Multiple Ch(

DERMATOLOGY

S. K. Goolamali, MD (Lond), FRCP
Consultant Dermatologist
Northwick Park Hospital
Harrow, Middlesex
England

Wolfe Publishing

Copyright © 1992 Mosby–Year Book Europe Ltd
Published in 1992 by Wolfe Publishing, an imprint of Mosby–Year
Book Europe Ltd
Printed by BPCC Hazells Ltd, Aylesbury, England
ISBN 0 7234 1769 5
For full details of all Mosby–Year Book Europe Ltd titles please write
to Mosby–Year Book Ltd, Brook House, 2–16 Torrington Place,
London WC1E 7LT, England.

CONTENTS

To all those who recognize Dermatology as more than skin deep – this book is dedicated

PREFACE

The curriculum of many medical schools worldwide suffers from insufficient time being made available to the less glamorous specialties, such as Dermatology. The consequence is that a significant number of students and doctors find skin diseases a mystery enmeshed in Latin or Greek terminology, or alternatively assume that every eruption which threatens to itch is scabies! Community studies, in both England and the United States, suggest that at the very least the prevalence of some form of skin pathology in the population is 20%. If one in five of the populace is likely to suffer a skin condition, it behoves every medical practitioner to learn to separate the macule from the papule.

This book, however, is not a textbook of Dermatology. It cannot and does not purport to replace several excellent textbooks which provide the structured teaching required to grasp the fundamentals and enjoy the minutiae of the specialty. Its aims are threefold. The first is to introduce students and non-dermatologists to the concept that the skin may reflect internal disease. The second is to provide packaged information on selected subjects to help the reader consolidate previously acquired facts or identify subjects that require further in-depth reading. The third is to offer a selection of questions randomly formulated to allow practice for those examinations where multiple choice questions are used routinely.

There are 10 papers, each of which gives 20 questions. Each question is composed of a stem followed by a variable number of statements. Any number of statements may be correct. The reader is invited to identify both 'true' and 'false' statements. For those who wish to assess their skills, a correct answer, which may be either 'true' or 'false', gains one mark, while an incorrect answer loses a mark. No marks are awarded for 'don't know'. The answers given for each question relate to those statements that are true only. As with all such tests, it is vital to read the question carefully and not to guess at the answer.

The references after each paper are chosen as a guide to further reading and should be considered to be of a core status rather than the very latest discourse on the subject. The information in this book has been ratified whenever possible by reference to three different sources. Those texts which have been particularly useful are listed under 'Selected Bibliography'.

QUESTIONS

PAPER ONE

1.1. **Lichenoid eruptions may result from treatment with:**

A   chloroquine
B   chlorothiazide
C   mepacrine
D   methyldopa
E   amiphenazole

1.2. **Dermatomyositis**

A   a significant proportion of adult patients have an underlying neoplasm
B   weakness of the limb muscles is mainly proximal
C   in children it is usually associated with a hypernephroma
D   the majority of patients with calcinosis are females
E   neoplasm when present usually precedes the dermatomyositis

1.3. **Sympathectomy is of recognised value in**

A   hyperhidrosis
B   cutis marmorata
C   thrombo-angiitis obliterans
D   phlebothrombosis
E   hypertensive (Martorell's) ulcer
F   mycetoma

1.4.   Match the following

A   Cullen's sign – miners; develop at sites of abrasions
B   Mitsuda reaction – sand flea; impregnated female, burrows
C   Collier's stripes – pellagra; dermatitis exacerbated with sunlight
D   Casal's necklace – psoralens; oil of Bergamot; pigmentation around the neck
E   Berloque dermatitis – leprosy-positive in tuberculoid type
F   'Jiggers' – bruising around the umbilicus; acute pancreatitis

1.5.   Erythema nodosum

A   nodules commonly affect the extensor aspects of the legs
B   ulceration of lesions occurs in a minority of cases
C   bilateral hilar lymphadenopathy, when associated, is diagnostic of sarcoidosis
D   a positive Kveim reaction excludes Crohn's disease as a possible cause
E   arthralgia is a commonly associated symptom, whatever the aetiology

1.6.   Pemphigus vulgaris

A   an essential abnormality is separation of epidermal cells from one another, or 'acantholysis'
B   oral mucosal lesions often precede skin lesions
C   large bullae that rupture with difficulty are characteristic
D   lesions usually heal with hyperpigmentation
E   autoantibodies to intercellular substance are found in the sera of affected patients
F   spontaneous remissions are common in patients with hypo-albuminaemia

1.7.   In the treatment of systemic lupus erythematosus (SLE)

A   a sunny climate is to be recommended
B   vitamin C in large doses can lead to resolution of the rash
C   phenylbutazone is the drug of choice for arthralgia, when present
D   antimalarials are particularly useful for photosensitivity
E   recent evidence suggests that thymectomy produces remission of the disease
F   erythrocyte sedimentation rate (ESR) is a satisfactory guide to progress

1.8.   Brucellosis

A   humans can be infected by ingestion of raw cow's milk
B   specific agglutinins in a titre of 1:320 or above is virtually diagnostic
C   a positive skin test with Brucella antigen is strong evidence of active infection
D   profuse nocturnal sweats are a common manifestation
E   contact with the secretions of an infected animal can give rise to local wealing

1.9.   Sarcoidosis

A   the most common neurological lesion is seventh cranial nerve palsy
B   the cutaneous forms predominantly affect females
C   diminished delayed hypersensitivity is characteristic
D   tubercle bacilli are not infrequently isolated from cutaneous lesions of sarcoid
E   corticosteroid therapy returns hypercalcaemia to normal values
F   the Kveim test is positive in the majority of patients with active disease

1.10.   Herpes simplex may present as

A   keratoconjunctivitis
B   vulvovaginitis
C   eczema herpeticum
D   meningo-encephalitis
E   gingivostomatitis

1.11. Reiter's disease

A   may develop after bacillary dysentery
B   skin lesions once present are lifelong stigmata
C   occurs mainly in young male adults
D   keratoderma blennorrhagicum is usually limited to the extensor surfaces of the body
E   typically presents as urethritis
F   arthritis commonly affects joints of the lower limbs
G   deep vein thrombophlebitis is a recognised complication

1.12. Sunlight is a recognised aggravating factor in

A   systemic lupus erythematosus
B   dermatomyositis
C   porphyria cutanea tarda
D   pellagra
E   phaeochromocytoma
F   rosacea

1.13. Livedo reticularis is a known cutaneous association of

A   rheumatoid arthritis
B   rheumatic fever
C   myxoedema
D   thrombocythaemia
E   polyarteritis nodosa
F   cryoglobulinaemia

1.14. Scleroderma-like syndromes have been described with

A   bleomycin therapy
B   pentazocine abuse
C   manufacture of polyvinyl chloride (PVC)
D   ingestion of denatured rapeseed oil
E   juvenile rheumatoid arthritis

1.15. Photosensitivity may be produced by

A   aspirin
B   halogenated salicylanilides
C   demeclocycline hydrochloride
D   oil of Bergamot
E   furocoumarins
F   tolbutamide
G   chlorpromazine

1.16. Localised morphoea

A   may be provoked by local trauma
B   may be exacerbated by pregnancy
C   expected natural history is towards spontaneous resolution
D   spina bifida is a common associated abnormality
E   produces frontoparietal lesions that may result in an abnormal electroencephalogram tracing

1.17. Choose the correct statement/s: Yaws,

A   may be transmitted from mother to child *in utero*
B   plantar lesions are common
C   causal spirochaete *Treponema pertenue* can penetrate intact skin
D   multiple cutaneous granulomata are characteristic
E   periostitis is known to occur in association with infectious skin lesions
F   in typical untreated cases the treponemal immobilisation test is positive

1.18. Cutaneous manifestations of infectious mononucleosis include

A   jaundice
B   pinpoint petechiae at the junction of hard and soft palates
C   herpes simplex
D   herpes zoster
E   regular pitting of the nails
F   purpura

1.19. Chronic venous ulceration is often associated with

A   Paget's disease of bone
B   subcutaneous calcification
C   periostitis of underlying bone
D   malignant change in an ulcer
E   lymphoedema

1.20. Dermatological manifestations of rheumatoid arthritis include

A   painless infarcts around the nails
B   punched-out leg ulcers
C   increased skin fragility
D   subcutaneous nodules
E   pyoderma gangrenosum

PAPER TWO

2.1. Erythema multiforme may be triggered off by

A   vaccinia
B   pregnancy
C   radiotherapy
D   mycoplasma infection
E   herpes simplex
F   phenylbutazone
G   barbiturates

2.2. Cutaneous manifestations of cirrhosis of the liver include

A   palmar erythema
B   spider naevi
C   loss of axillary and pubic hair
D   gynaecomastia
E   white nails
F   generalised hyperpigmentation
G   xanthomata

2.3. The incidence of premature greying of hair is increased in

A   thyrotoxicosis
B   dystrophia myotonica
C   progeria
D   kala-azar
E   tuberous sclerosis

2.4. **Macroglossia may be found in the following**

A   Pierre Robin syndrome
B   cretinism
C   acromegaly
D   angioneurotic oedema
E   primary amyloidosis
F   median rhomboid glossitis

2.5. **Viral infections that involve the oral mucosa include**

A   herpes simplex
B   varicella
C   herpes zoster
D   hand, foot, and mouth disease
E   herpangina

2.6. **Hypermelanosis is a feature of the following hereditary syndromes**

A   Waardenburg's syndrome
B   Peutz–Jeghers syndrome
C   Chediak–Higashi syndrome
D   Albright's syndrome
E   xeroderma pigmentosum
F   incontinentia pigmenti
G   Gaucher's disease

2.7. **Erythroderma**

A   lymphadenopathy is a common feature
B   hypothermia is a serious risk
C   steatorrhoea when associated usually responds to treatment of the skin alone
D   hepatic function is abnormal in most patients
E   cardiac output is usually decreased owing to an increased skin blood flow

2.8. **Specific cutaneous lesions and mental deficiency occur in**

A   epiloia
B   Darier's disease
C   phenylketonuria
D   Down's syndrome
E   Hartnup disease

2.9. **Cutaneous lesions associated with sarcoidosis include**

A   lupus pernio
B   subcutaneous nodules
C   erythema nodosum
D   scarring alopecia
E   thickened nails
F   fusiform swellings of the proximal interphalangeal joints

2.10. **Which of the following diseases is transmitted by mosquitos?**

A   bilharziasis
B   trypanosomiasis
C   yellow fever
D   filariasis
E   kala-azar
F   schistosomiasis
G   cysticercosis

2.11. **Malar flush is a recognised clinical sign in the following**

A   systemic lupus erythematosus (SLE)
B   rosacea
C   seborrhoeic dermatitis
D   mitral stenosis
E   scarlet fever
F   carcinoid
G   solar urticaria

2.12. **Diffuse alopecia is known to occur in**

A   Sheehan's syndrome
B   hypothyroidism
C   hyperthyroidism
D   hypoparathyroidism
E   homocystinuria
F   excessive consumption of Vitamin A
G   dystrophia myotonica
H   secondary syphilis

2.13. Arterial leg ulceration is a known complication of

A   diabetes
B   sickle-cell anaemia
C   hereditary spherocytosis
D   anterior tibial syndrome
E   barbiturate poisoning
F   Still's disease

2.14. Hypergammaglobulinaemia and cutaneous involvement may both be features of

A   Sjögren's syndrome
B   Hodgkin's disease
C   nephrotic syndrome
D   sarcoidosis
E   systemic lupus erythematosus
F   cirrhosis of the liver
G   ulcerative colitis

2.15. Hypertrichosis can be a prominent feature in

A   erythropoietic porphyria
B   Hurler's syndrome
C   pretibial myxoedema
D   anorexia nervosa
E   children on diphenylhydantoin therapy

2.16. Renal and cutaneous lesions as part of the same pathological process occur in the following

A   tuberous sclerosis
B   sickle-cell disease
C   hereditary haemorrhagic telangiectasia
D   systemic lupus erythematosus
E   erythema multiforme
F   polyarteritis nodosa

2.17. Onycholysis occurs in

A   lichen planus
B   Raynaud's disease
C   fungal infection
D   local trauma
E   myxoedema
F   psoriasis

2.18. **Cutaneous associations of thyrotoxicosis include**

A   xanthomata
B   clubbing
C   vitiligo
D   palmar erythema
E   hyperpigmentation
F   pretibial myxoedema
G   hypohidrosis

2.19. **Arterial insufficiency of the lower limbs may manifest itself as**

A   thin toe nails
B   intermittent claudication
C   reduced dorsalis pedis and posterior tibial pulses
D   punched-out ulcers over the ankles
E   paraesthesia in the toes
F   varicose veins

2.20. **Diabetes mellitus is a recognised complication of the following**

A   acromegaly
B   hyperparathyroidism
C   porphyria cutanea tarda
D   Cushing's syndrome
E   partial lipo-atrophy
F   haemochromatosis

PAPER THREE

3.1. **Pancreatic disease has the following cutaneous associations**

A   livedo reticularis
B   nodular fat necrosis
C   thrombophlebitis migrans
D   urticaria
E   bruise-like discolouration of the skin around the umbilicus

3.2. Purpura associated with fever occurs commonly in

A serum sickness
B polyarteritis nodosa
C Henoch–Schönlein purpura
D scurvy
E Takayasu's disease
F temporal arteritis

3.3. The head or neck is frequently involved in

A scabies
B impetigo contagiosa
C erysipelas
D recurrent herpes simplex
E Buerger's disease
F herpes zoster

3.4. Premenstrual exacerbation is often reported with

A acne vulgaris
B rosacea
C anogenital pruritus
D verruca vulgaris
E pityriasis capitis
F lupus erythematosus

3.5. Diseases associated with pyoderma gangrenosum include

A chronic myeloid leukaemia
B diabetes mellitus
C ulcerative colitis
D pustular psoriasis
E rheumatoid arthritis
F Crohn's disease

3.6. Telangiectasia is commonly found in the following

A scurvy
B steroid atrophy of the skin
C ataxia telangiectasia
D rosacea
E Rothmund–Thomson syndrome
F cirrhosis of the liver

3.7. **Skin disorders associated with diabetes mellitus include**

A   recurrent staphylococcal lesions
B   xanthoma diabeticorum
C   localised pruritus
D   acute dermatophytosis
E   rubeosis of the face
F   hyperhidrosis
G   alopecia

3.8. **In the newborn the following may present as lesions of the umbilicus**

A   hernia
B   talc granuloma
C   patent urachus
D   pyogenic granuloma
E   granulation tissue
F   undescended testis

3.9. **Angiomatous naevi of the skin may be associated with**

A   haemangiomatous involvement of underlying bone
B   thrombocytopenic purpura
C   retrolental fibroplasia
D   polycythaemia
E   angiomatosis of the retina and cerebellum

3.10. **Cutaneous changes associated with hypocalcaemia include**

A   widespread xeroderma
B   brittle nails
C   patchy alopecia of the scalp
D   hypopigmented plaques
E   impetigo 'herpetiformis'
F   Candida infection of nail folds

3.11. **Features of acute graft-versus-host disease include**

A   hepatitis
B   purpura
C   diarrhoea
D   lymphocytopenia
E   toxic epidermal necrolysis
F   scleroderma
G   lichen planus-like lesions

3.12. **Dermatoses that commonly affect the anogenital region are**

A   candidiasis
B   keratoderma blenorrhagica
C   pediculosis
D   hidradenitis suppurativa
E   erythrasma
F   pemphigoid

3.13. **The oral cavity may be involved in the following metabolic disorders**

A   primary amyloidosis
B   Gaucher's disease
C   diabetes mellitus
D   lipoid proteinosis
E   Hand–Schüller–Christian disease

3.14. **Clinical features of lepromatous leprosy include**

A   saddle nose deformity
B   loose (one or both) upper central incisor teeth
C   leonine facies
D   ulceration of legs
E   testicular atrophy
F   gynaecomastia
G   erythema nodosum
H   involvement of 8th, 9th and 10th cranial nerves

3.15. **Increased sensitivity to ultraviolet radiation is a feature of**

A   oculocutaneous albinism
B   acute intermittent porphyria
C   phenylketonuria
D   vitiligo
E   Chediak–Higashi syndrome

3.16. **Hypopigmentation of skin may result from**

A   dithranol treatment of psoriasis
B   leprosy
C   pityriasis alba
D   pinta
E   chronic urticaria
F   herpes zoster

3.17. Changes suggestive of malignancy in pigmented naevi are

A   presence of new pigment around a naevus
B   development of uneven surface pigmentation
C   sudden enlargement of a previously quiescent 'mole'
D   increase in hair in a hairy naevus
E   ulceration in a naevus

3.18. The following are recognised in the aetiology of erythema nodosum

A   sarcoidosis
B   tuberculosis
C   streptococcal infection
D   Behçet's disease
E   cat scratch fever
F   Yersinia infection
G   measles

3.19. Blistering lesions in the mouth may be a result of

A   Darier's disease
B   pemphigoid
C   erythema multiforme
D   benign mucous membrane pemphigoid
E   dermatitis herpetiformis
F   pemphigus vulgaris
G   lichen planus

3.20. Lesions over the soles of the feet may be present in

A   papular secondary syphilis
B   solar dermatitis
C   contact dermatitis
D   *Trichophyton rubrum* infection
E   psoriasis
F   cutaneous larva migrans

PAPER FOUR

4.1.   Pregnancy is known to predispose to

A   Candida vulvovaginitis
B   systemic lupus erythematosus
C   spider telangiectases
D   herpes gestationis
E   sarcoidosis
F   pigmentation
G   palmar erythema
H   pruritus

4.2.   Which of the following is associated with tabes dorsalis?

A   posterior column degeneration
B   abdominal 'crises'
C   optic atrophy
D   gumma formation
E   trophic joint changes
F   irregular pupil which reacts to light but not to accommodation
G   loss of deep pain sensation

4.3.   Abnormal jejunal biopsy is a feature of

A   dermatitis herpetiformis
B   tropical sprue
C   amyloidosis
D   giardiasis
E   Whipple's disease
F   coeliac disease

4.4.   Whitening of the nails may be a sign in

A   arsenical poisoning
B   Darier's disease
C   lymphoedema
D   chronic hypo-albuminaemia
E   *Pseudomonas pyocyanea* infection of the nails
F   cirrhosis of the liver

4.5. **Rocky Mountain spotted fever**

A   the causative organism is *Rickettsia prowazekii*
B   transmission from human-to-human is by the bite of an infected louse
C   rash appears 3–4 days after onset of fever
D   bilateral symmetrical purpura of the palms and soles is typical
E   disseminated intravascular coagulation may complicate disease
F   diagnosis is best made by direct immunofluorescence of a skin biopsy

4.6. **Rash associated with Still's disease (juvenile rheumatoid arthritis) has the following features**

A   lesions increase in size with each recurrence
B   lasts only a few hours at a time
C   characteristically appears with an increase in the temperature of the patient
D   may occur intermittently for years
E   more frequent in girls
F   more common in patients with associated lymphadenopathy

4.7. **Rubella contracted in the first trimester of pregnancy may cause in the newborn**

A   oesophageal atresia
B   thrombocytopenic purpura
C   cataracts
D   patent ductus arteriosus
E   microcephaly
F   hepatosplenomegaly

4.8. **Disorders that commonly exhibit both cutaneous and neurological signs include**

A   Refsum's syndrome
B   vitamin A deficiency
C   homocystinuria
D   acrodynia
E   Behçet's disease
F   kuru
G   Lesch–Nyhan syndrome

4.9. Sjögren's syndrome

A   keratoconjunctivitis sicca is a common feature
B   rheumatoid arthritis is frequently associated
C   tear secretion is usually significantly reduced
D   anogenital pruritus is an occasional presenting symptom
E   splenic enlargement is a recognised manifestation
F   antinuclear antibodies are present in the majority of cases

4.10. Which of the following are accepted clinical features of idiopathic haemochromatosis?

A   Addisonian-like pigmentation
B   sparing of mucous membranes
C   diabetes mellitus
D   hepatosplenomegaly
E   sexual impotence
F   greater frequency in women
G   resistant congestive cardiac failure

4.11. Subcutaneous nodules are a recognised feature of

A   erythema induratum
B   pityriasis versicolor
C   erythema nodosum
D   Behçet's disease
E   polyarteritis nodosa
F   Gaucher's disease
G   pretibial myoedema

4.12. Lichen planus

A   mucous membrane lesions uncommonly involve the tongue
B   typical lesions are shiny papules with overlying Wickham's striae
C   annular lesions are common on the glans penis
D   thinning of the nail plate is the commonest nail change
E   alopecia as a complication is usually non-scarring
F   lichen planus-like eruptions may result from processing colour film

4.13. Dangers of oral corticosteroid therapy include

A   activation of tuberculosis
B   decreased blood viscosity
C   increase in incidence of gastric ulceration
D   hypokalaemia
E   osteomalacia
F   induction of bacteriaemia
G   delayed healing of wounds

4.14. Clinical manifestations of hypopituitarism include

A   cold intolerance
B   absence of pubic and axillary hair
C   mild cutaneous hyperpigmentation
D   prominent muscle wasting
E   fine wrinkling around the eyes
F   genital atrophy
G   amelioration of pre-existing diabetes mellitus

4.15. Fever and typically an erythematous eruption are found in

A   measles
B   infectious mononucleosis
C   Kaposi's varicelliform eruption
D   toxic shock syndrome
E   toxic epidermal necrolysis
F   hand, foot, and mouth disease
G   Lyme disease

4.16. Scarlet fever

A   'strawberry tongue' is commonly seen by the third day of illness
B   a positive Hess' sign is found in a majority of cases
C   rash appears on the second day
D   a positive Dick test indicates that the patient is immune
E   myocarditis is a recognised complication

4.17. Long-term immunity commonly follows an unmodified attack of

A   mumps
B   quartan malaria
C   rubella
D   orf
E   erysipelas
F   measles
G   yellow fever

4.18. Which of the following can cause hypopituitarism?

A   syphilis
B   Hodgkin's disease
C   basal skull fracture
D   sarcoidosis
E   scleroderma
F   Hand–Schüller–Christian disease
G   primary aldosteronism
H   chromophobe adenoma

4.19. Secondary syphilis

A   skin lesions are usually bilateral and symmetrical
B   vesiculobullous lesions are a frequent manifestation in adults
C   'moth-eaten' alopecia is characteristic
D   mucous patches when present involve the mouth alone
E   loss of eyelashes may be a feature
F   *Treponema pallidum* can be isolated from a secondary skin lesion

4.20. Features of the Sturge–Weber syndrome include

A   unilateral 'port-wine' facial naevus
B   absence of oral manifestations
C   hemiplegia of the side opposite to the unilateral naevus
D   mental retardation
E   convolutional calcification of the cerebral cortex
F   hypercalcaemia

PAPER FIVE

5.1. **Underlying malignancy may be heralded by**

A   diffuse hyperpigmentation of the skin
B   Paget's disease of the nipple
C   acanthosis nigricans
D   blue–green pigmentation of the finger tips
E   dermatomyositis
F   herpes zoster

5.2. **Trophic ulceration may occur in**

A   tabes dorsalis
B   sciatic nerve injury
C   diabetes mellitus
D   spinal dysraphism
E   syringomyelia
F   leprosy
G   *Clostridium botulinum* infection

5.3. **Napkin eruption in an infant may be due to**

A   seborrhoeic eczema
B   miliaria
C   juvenile pemphigoid
D   petroleum jelly application
E   acrodermatitis enteropathica
F   Letterer–Siwe disease

5.4. **Hyperpigmentation may be prominent in**

A   acromegaly
B   tinea versicolor
C   Cushing's syndrome
D   haemochromatosis
E   pregnancy
F   scleroderma

5.5. *Candida albicans*

A   can exist as a saprophyte in healthy adults
B   untreated diabetes mellitus predisposes to Candida infection
C   fluoresces green under Wood's light
D   increased candidiasis in hypoparathyroidism
E   may cause endocarditis after vascular surgery
F   is a frequent secondary pathogen in napkin rash

5.6. Cold may aggravate

A   cutis marmorata
B   chilblains
C   Raynaud's phenomenon
D   herpes simplex
E   erythema ab igne
F   hyperhidrosis

5.7. Phenylketonuria

A   a manifestation is infantile eczema
B   phenylalanine hydroxylase is usually absent
C   mental deficiency is a common sequel
D   therapy involves a diet low in phenylalanine
E   electroencephalogram is abnormal in the majority

5.8. Known side effects of oral contraceptives include

A   hirsutes
B   chloasma
C   photosensitivity
D   diffuse alopecia
E   herpes gestationis
F   genital candidiasis

5.9. The following dermatoses have a predilection for the hands

A   herpes zoster
B   vitiligo
C   anthrax
D   lichen sclerosus
E   erysipeloid
F   pompholyx

5.10. The following are inherited as autosomal dominant traits

A   tuberous sclerosis
B   Peutz–Jeghers syndrome
C   hereditary haemorrhagic telangiectasia
D   diabetes mellitus
E   psoriasis
F   acne vulgaris

5.11. Linear lesions are commonly seen in

A   sporotrichosis
B   tinea circinata
C   epidermal naevi
D   molluscum contagiosum
E   morphoea in children
F   erythema annulare centrifugum

5.12. Human immunodeficiency virus (HIV)

A   is characterised by life-long persistence in its host
B   the acute infection can induce a glandular fever-like illness
C   the majority of symptomatic patients have decreased numbers of T-helper cells usually below 100/mm^3
D   the interval between acquisition of HIV and onset of AIDS may be several years
E   transmission is mainly by blood and semen
F   transmission through artificial insemination has occurred

5.13. Gynaecomastia may occur with

A   bronchial carcinoma
B   cholera
C   spironolactone administration
D   chronic liver disease
E   malnutrition
F   testicular tumour
G   digitalis therapy

5.14. An increased incidence of vitiligo is found in

A   diabetes mellitus
B   Addison's disease
C   thyrotoxicosis
D   pernicious anaemia
E   alopecia areata
F   tinea versicolor

5.15. Clubbing may be found with

A   metastatic cancer to the thorax
B   cirrhosis
C   ulcerative colitis
D   coarctation of the aorta
E   thyrotoxicosis
F   bronchogenic carcinoma

5.16. Genital ulceration may be a result of

A   Peyronie's disease
B   *Candida albicans*
C   herpes simplex
D   Reiter's disease
E   pemphigus vulgaris
F   Behçet's disease
G   Stevens–Johnson syndrome

5.17. Scarring alopecia may result from

A   metastases to the scalp
B   discoid lupus erythematosus
C   sarcoidosis
D   lichen planus
E   alopecia areata
F   cyclophosphamide therapy

5.18. Neurofibromatosis

A   café-au-lait spots are the most common disturbances of pigmentation
B   a pathognomonic sign is the presence of freckle-like pigmentation in axillae
C   the commonest solitary intracranial tumour is an optic nerve glioma
D   inheritance is as a sex-linked recessive trait
E   neurofibroma may undergo sarcomatous transformation
F   endocrine abnormalities may be associated

5.19. Generalised pruritus can be a feature of

A   trichinosis
B   lymphatic leukaemia
C   drug reactions
D   chronic renal failure
E   Hodgkin's disease
F   biliary cirrhosis
G   iron deficiency

5.20. Oral mucosa can be involved in

A   lichen planus
B   Peutz–Jeghers syndrome
C   Addison's disease
D   discoid lupus erythematosus
E   pemphigoid
F   infection with viral warts

PAPER SIX

6.1. Pyoderma gangrenosum

A   high protein diet normally leads to resolution of the lesions
B   characteristic lesion is an irregular ulcer with a necrotic base
C   occurs in rheumatoid arthritis
D   In ulcerative colitis lesions tend to parallel the activity of the bowel disease
E   may occur in patients who are otherwise in good health

6.2. Viral diseases characterised by cutaneous lesions include

A   rabies
B   molluscum contagiosum
C   rubella
D   Rocky Mountain spotted fever
E   orf
F   impetigo contagiosa
G   poliomyelitis

6.3. Signs of late congenital syphilis include

A rhagades
B perforation of hard palate
C maldevelopment of permanent central incisors
D eighth nerve deafness
E bowing of the tibia
F paresis
G interstitial keratitis

6.4. Typhoid fever

A positive blood cultures occur in the first week of illness
B 'rose spots' usually appear in the second week of the disease
C intestinal haemorrhage commonly occurs on the third or fourth day of illness
D chloramphenicol therapy significantly decreases the incidence of chronic carriers
E effective prophylaxis is ensured by immunisation every third year

6.5. Cutaneous manifestations of HIV disease include

A seborrhoeic eczema
B herpes zoster
C itchy folliculitis
D oral hairy leukoplakia
E sulphonamide-induced drug reaction
F molluscum contagiosum infection

6.6. Lupus vulgaris

A occurs as a post-primary infection
B characteristic lesion is a plaque composed of 'apple jelly' coloured nodules
C *Mycobacterium tuberculosis* is cultured from skin lesions in the majority of patients
D conjunctival mucosa may be involved
E squamous cell epithelioma can develop in affected skin

6.7.   Raynaud's phenomenon

A   the hands are affected more often than the feet
B   typical attacks consist of cyanosis, erythema, and pallor successively
C   severe cases may result in pulp atrophy
D   acrocyanosis is distinguished by the absence of the paroxysmal pallor
E   with asymmetrical involvement of the digits a cervical rib is often the cause
F   oesophageal aperistalsis may occur in association

6.8.   A positive test for rheumatoid factor is an expected finding in

A   ochronosis
B   Sjögren's syndrome
C   agammaglobulinaemia
D   kala-azar
E   systemic lupus erythematosus
F   psoriatic arthritis
G   Felty's syndrome
H   Reiter's disease

6.9.   Psoriasis

A   can be produced experimentally in animals
B   streptococcal infection is a frequent provoking agent in children
C   measles often improves or clears the disease temporarily
D   may first appear after parturition
E   generalised pustular psoriasis can be precipitated by hypocalcaemia

6.10.   Glucagonoma syndrome

A   is caused by an islet cell tumour of the pancreas
B   patients typically affected are grossly obese
C   skin eruption resembles toxic epidermal necrolysis
D   normochromic anaemia is common
E   antibiotic therapy usually clears the rash
F   diabetes is often associated

6.11. Purpura is usually non-thrombocytopenic in

A Cushing's syndrome
B senile purpura
C incompatible transfusion reaction
D cachexia
E pernicious anaemia
F corticosteroid therapy

6.12. Cutaneous features of Cushing's syndrome include

A hirsutism
B tinea versicolor
C plethoric facies
D purple abdominal striae
E mottled hyperpigmentation over the trunk
F acneiform eruption over the face
G scarring alopecia
H easy bruising

6.13. Secondary amyloidosis is a recognised complication of

A hidradenitis suppurativa
B lepromatous leprosy
C epidermolysis bullosa
D recurrent cystic acne
E long-standing osteoarthritis
F chronic rheumatoid arthritis

6.14. Recognised manifestations of systemic mastocytosis include

A skin lesions
B dermographism
C extra-pyramidal signs
D bone lesions
E peptic ulcers
F hepatosplenomegaly

6.15. Porphyria cutanea tarda

A often associated with excessive consumption of alcohol
B acute attacks may be provoked by barbiturates
C hepatomegaly is common
D scars on the dorsa of the hands are an expected finding
E serum iron level is frequently elevated
F faecal protoporphyrin excretion is usually found to be increased

6.16. Common features of kwashiorkor are

A   retarded growth
B   pitting oedema of the lower limbs
C   alopecia
D   constipation
E   hyperalbuminaemia
F   pellagra-like dermatosis

6.17. Syphilis in pregnancy

A   the longer the duration of untreated infection before pregnancy, the less likely it is that the fetus will be stillborn
B   adequate treatment of the mother before the 18th week of pregnancy usually prevents infection of the fetus
C   usually causes a stillbirth rather than an abortion
D   after the 18th week of gestation, the placenta acts as an effective barrier against penicillin

6.18. Rubella

A   rash occurs on the first or second day of the illness
B   suboccipital lymphadenopathy is usually present
C   the earliest spots emerge on the face
D   in adults a complication may be arthritis
E   Koplik's spots as found in measles may be present
F   absence of rash is particularly common in young children

6.19. Drugs that significantly result in hyperpigmentation as a side effect include

A   chlorpromazine
B   aspirin
C   barbiturates
D   busulfan
E   hydantoin
F   chloroquine

6.20. Precocious puberty may be a manifestation of

A   tuberous sclerosis
B   neurofibromatosis
C   Stein–Leventhal syndrome
D   craniopharyngioma
E   cryptorchidism
F   McCune–Albright's syndrome
G   Klinefelter's syndrome

PAPER SEVEN

7.1. **The following drugs may cause a lupus erythematosus-like syndrome**

A procainamide
B isoniazid
C aspirin
D hydralazine
E anticonvulsants

7.2. **Kaposi's sarcoma in AIDS**

A early histological changes may be detected in clinically unaffected skin
B in most cases its course is insidious
C skin lesions are the usual presentation
D visceral lesions are rare
E skin lesions may develop at sites of trauma (Köebner's phenomenon)
F the tumour is not responsive to radiotherapy

7.3. **Palmar erythema may be found in**

A rheumatoid arthritis
B pregnancy
C families as a dominant trait
D cinchonism
E cirrhosis of the liver
F erythroderma

7.4. **Griseofulvin**

A absorption is increased if taken after food
B is fungicidal rather than fungistatic
C diminishes the anticoagulant effect of warfarin
D has no activity against bacteria
E blood levels are reduced if given simultaneously with phenobarbitone

7.5. **Secondary xanthomatosis is known to occur in**

A hypothyroidism
B nephrotic syndrome
C multiple myeloma
D acute intermittent porphyria
E haemochromatosis
F hyperparathyroidism
G primary biliary cirrhosis

7.6. **Causes of Raynaud's phenomemon include**

A ergot intoxication
B lupus erythematosus
C systemic sclerosis
D 'pill rolling' movements in Parkinsonism
E dermatomyositis
F piano playing
G pregnancy

7.7. **Measles infection may result in**

A an improvement of eczema
B remission of Hodgkin's disease
C remission of leukaemia
D a transient suppression of the tuberculin reaction
E demyelinating encephalomyelitis
F activation of pre-existing tuberculosis

7.8. **Acneiform eruptions can be caused by**

A co-trimoxazole
B iodides
C isoniazid
D tetracycline
E ACTH

7.9. **Leg ulceration may occur in**

A brucellosis
B leprosy
C leishmaniasis
D ulcerative colitis
E necrobiosis lipoidica diabeticorum
F sickle cell anaemia

7.10. Grouped lesions are often present in

A   insect bites
B   urticaria
C   herpes zoster
D   discoid lupus erythematosus
E   Campbell de Morgan spots
F   dematitis herpetiformis

7.11. Clinical signs of systemic sclerosis are

A   'beaking' of the nose
B   radial furrowing around the mouth
C   swelling of the hands
D   atrophy of terminal phalanges
E   short stature
F   mat-like telangiectasia over the face

7.12. Köebner's phenomenon may be seen in

A   viral warts
B   lichen planus
C   eczema
D   psoriasis
E   scabies

7.13. Cutaneous manifestations of systemic lupus erythematosus include

A   photosensitivity
B   chronic discoid lupus erythematosus
C   telangiectatic erythema over the hands
D   purpura
E   'butterfly' eruption over the face
F   scarring alopecia
G   leg ulcer

7.14. Measles

A   Koplik's spots appear on the buccal mucosa on the second day of illness
B   the rash usually involves the palms and soles
C   once the eruption has appeared the patient is no longer infectious
D   a morbilliform rash appears on the third or fourth day
E   bullous lesions may occur in severe forms of the disease

7.15. Bone involvement is a recognised manifestation of

A idiopathic calcinosis cutis
B psoriasis
C Reiter's disease
D tertiary syphilis
E Albright's syndrome
F pemphigus vulgaris

7.16. Wood's light

A is ultraviolet light emitted through a nickel oxide filter
B shows a coral-pink fluorescence with erythrasma
C produces a brilliant green fluorescence with *Microsporum audouinii* infection
D is useful in the treatment of porphyria cutanea tarda
E fluoresces tinea versicolor blue

7.17. Both the skin and eyes can be involved in

A acne vulgaris
B rosacea
C discoid lupus erythematosus
D Crohn's disease
E Behçet's syndrome
F bullous pemphigoid

7.18. Contraindications to immunisation are

A previous smallpox infection
B pregnancy
C patient on immunosuppressive treatment
D leukaemia
E infantile eczema

7.19. Important criteria for the diagnosis of systemic lupus erythematosus (SLE) are

A an erythrocyte sedimentation rate of 20 mm or more in the first hour
B a rash compatible with SLE
C a white cell count below 5000 cells/mm^3
D a positive antinuclear antibody test
E a positive test for rheumatoid factor
F retinal changes

7.20. Tuberculin test

A   the size of reaction may be diminished if the patient is on systemic steroids

B   a negative result excludes *Mycobacterium tuberculosis* infection

C   an induration of greater than 10 mm after 5 tuberculin units (TU) is virtually diagnostic of *M. tuberculosis* infection

D   a negative result is commonly found in sarcoidosis

E   the Heaf test is more likely to be negative than the Mantoux test

PAPER EIGHT

8.1. Natural history of syphilis

A   a chancre may develop up to 3 months after infection

B   serologic tests are usually positive when the chancre first appears

C   the interval between the primary lesion and the secondary eruption is usually 6–8 weeks

D   cutaneous relapse can occur after the secondary eruption has healed

E   untreated patients invariably develop symptomatic tertiary syphilis

F   seroreversal indicates spontaneous cure

8.2. Blue sclerae may occur in

A   Ehlers–Danlos syndrome

B   Marfan's syndrome

C   incontinentia pigmenti

D   Addison's disease

E   malaria

F   osteogenesis imperfecta

8.3. Albinos

A   excessive lanugo hair is common
B   inheritance is commonly as an autosomal recessive
C   photophobia is a frequent finding
D   increased susceptibility to skin cancer
E   there is an increased light sensitivity
F   patchy pigmentation may develop in skin exposed to light

8.4. Leukaemia

A   green facial tumor ('chloroma') is pathognomonic
B   specific cutaneous lesions are identical to those of malignant lymphomas
C   ulceration of skin lesions is commonest in monocytic leukaemia
D   leukaemic infiltration of facial skin may simulate rosacea
E   a biopsy of leukaemic infiltrate is diagnostic of cell type

8.5. Diseases that affect both the skin and intestine include

A   blind loop syndrome
B   hereditary angioedema
C   systemic amyloidosis
D   Crohn's disease
E   Cushing's disease
F   typhoid fever

8.6. Pigmentation of the nails can be a feature of

A   chloroquine therapy
B   Wilson's disease (hepato-lenticular degeneration)
C   vitamin B_{12} deficiency
D   pinta
E   nail–patella syndrome
F   argyria

8.7. The following vesiculo-bullous conditions are significantly associated with cancer

A   impetigo
B   erythema multiforme
C   bullous papular urticaria
D   dermatitis herpetiformis-like eruptions
E   epidermolysis bullosa
F   pompholyx

8.8. Peutz–Jeghers syndrome

A   transmission is as a recessive trait
B   brown–black lentigines usually occur on the lips
C   the majority show buccal pigmentation
D   increased incidence of hare-lip
E   jejunal polyps may be found

8.9. Increased sweating is characteristically associated with

A   mucoviscidosis
B   thyrotoxicosis
C   atropine poisoning
D   familial dysautonomia
E   destructive lesions of the hypothalamus
F   hypoglycaemia

8.10. Tuberous sclerosis

A   earliest cutaneous manifestation is adenoma sebaceum
B   periungual fibromata are a recognised association
C   X-ray may show lytic lesions in the phalanges
D   epilepsy usually begins after puberty
E   renal tumours are a common occurrence
F   retinal phakomata are found in a minority of cases

8.11. Periorbital oedema may be a conspicuous sign in

A   carcinoid syndrome
B   Chagas' disease
C   progeria
D   hereditary angio-oedema
E   trichinosis
F   erysipelas of the face

8.12. An increased frequency of a specific human leucocyte antigen has been reported in

A   Hodgkin's disease
B   malignant melanoma
C   adult coeliac disease
D   Sjögren's syndrome
E   Behçet's disease
F   pemphigus vulgaris

8.13. Fixed eruptions are commonly attributed to

A   griseofulvin
B   quinine
C   cimetidine
D   sulphonamides
E   gold
F   phenolphthalein

8.14. McCune–Albright's syndrome

A   may present as precocious puberty in females
B   pigmentation is most prominent on the side with most severe bone involvement
C   osseous cysts occur in long bones
D   pathological fractures are common
E   hyperthyroidism is frequently associated
F   asymmetrical skin pigmentation appears early in life

8.15. Malignant changes may be seen in

A   first-degree burns
B   radiodermatitis
C   xeroderma pigmentosum
D   lupus vulgaris
E   lentigo maligna

8.16. Urticaria has been attributed to

A   dental caries
B   arsenic intoxication
C   superficial fungus infection
D   occult malignancy
E   Candida hypersensitivity
F   systemic lupus erythematosus

8.17. Pseudoxanthoma elasticum

A   yellow papules over the body folds are characteristic
B   angioid streaks are an ocular hallmark
C   peripheral pulses may be absent
D   retinal haemorrhages are a recognised complication
E   postural hypotension is common
F   a significant association is with Paget's disease of bone
G   recurrent gastro-intestinal haemorrhage may occur

8.18. Superficial thrombophlebitis may result from

A butazolidine therapy
B prolonged immobilisation
C debility
D cancer of the pancreas
E pulmonary embolism
F trauma

8.19. Psoriatic arthritis

A skin lesions precede arthritis in the majority of cases
B rheumatoid-type nodules do not occur
C the classic form affects the distal interphalangeal joints
D spinal involvement may be clinically silent
E nail dystrophy is uncommon in the 'arthritis mutilans' type
F conjunctivitis is reported to occur in 20% of patients

8.20. Hodgkin's disease is significantly associated with

A generalised pruritus
B acquired ichthyosis
C exfoliative dermatitis
D lichen planus
E jaundice
F hyperpigmentation

PAPER NINE

9.1. In typical cases, diagnosis can often be made by examination of the face alone in

A cretinism
B Fallot's tetralogy
C Down's syndrome
D myasthenia gravis
E polycythaemia rubra vera
F tabes dorsalis
G advanced Wilson's disease

9.2. Ehlers–Danlos syndrome

A   hyperextensibility of the joints is a feature
B   there is an increased skin fragility
C   hypertelorism is common
D   presentation may be as 'spontaneous' pneumothorax
E   there is an increased frequency of hiatus hernia
F   a recognised complication is congenital hip dislocation

9.3. Acanthosis nigricans

A   may precede an internal malignancy
B   commonly affects the neck and flexures
C   is a recognised marker of gastric carcinoma
D   can be inherited as an autosomal dominant trait
E   may occur in acromegaly
F   has a known association with obesity

9.4. Carcinoid syndrome

A   cardiac involvement is predominantly left-sided
B   a facial flush with a violaceous hue is produced
C   skin lesions similar to pellagra may be caused
D   with appendiceal carcinoid skin signs are common
E   a malignant carcinoid typically develops from a primary tumour of the ileum
F   urinary 5-hydroxyindoleacetic acid is usually increased

9.5. Hartnup disease

A   tyrosinase deficiency is a basic defect
B   pellagra-like rash is characteristic
C   ataxia may develop in association with rash
D   there is an increased sensitivity to light
E   aminoaciduria is a persistent biochemical abnormality

9.6. Cutaneous metastases

A   distribution is usually centrifugal
B   the patient usually dies within 3–6 months of onset
C   may occur up to 15 years after surgery for breast cancer
D   the scalp is a favourite site for metastases from the lung
E   renal carcinoma may cause epulis-like lesions in the mouth
F   in prostatic cancer can occur in a zoster-like distribution over the flank

9.7. Hair loss may be caused by

A   cyclophosphamide
B   tetracycline
C   the contraceptive pill
D   phenytoin
E   heparin

9.8. Mycosis fungoides

A   is a systemic fungal infection
B   may present with pruritus
C   lymphadenopathy is common in advanced disease
D   lymphomatous involvement of viscera occurs
E   secondary infection is a frequent cause of death
F   tests for delayed hypersensitivity abnormal in early disease

9.9. Leukaemic infiltration of the skin

A   commonly involves the palms and soles
B   may arise in scars
C   is more common over the trunk in myeloid leukaemia
D   can simulate a fungal infection
E   may produce a leonine facies

9.10. Pruritus may be the presenting symptom of

A   obstructive liver disease
B   leprosy
C   polycythaemia rubra vera
D   multiple myeloma
E   thyrotoxicosis
F   alopecia areata

9.11. Hereditary haemorrhagic telangiectasia

A   anaemia when present is usually due to malabsorption
B   cutaneous telangiectasia characteristically increase in number with age
C   pulmonary arteriovenous fistulae are a recognised feature
D   gastric mucosa is often involved
E   the bleeding time is usually abnormal
F   may present as recurrent epistaxis

9.12. **Drugs known to aggravate hepatic porphyria include**

A   oral contraceptives
B   sulphonamides
C   methyldopa
D   griseofulvin
E   penicillin
F   aspirin

9.13. **Enlargement of the forehead in children may occur in**

A   rickets
B   Pierre Robin syndrome
C   hydrocephalus
D   congenital syphilis
E   Paget's disease of bone
F   haematoma

9.14. **Both oesophageal dysfunction and skin disease may occur in**

A   achalasia
B   dermatomyositis
C   diabetes mellitus
D   candidiasis
E   systemic sclerosis
F   acute Chagas' disease

9.15. **An increased incidence of ampicillin rash occurs in**

A   infectious mononucleosis
B   viral infections of the respiratory tract
C   coeliac disease
D   cytomegalovirus mononucleosis
E   lipoid proteinosis
F   lymphatic leukaemia

9.16. **Side effects of Dapsone include**

A   methaemoglobinaemia
B   fixed drug eruption
C   haemolytic anaemia
D   photosensitivity
E   peripheral neuropathy
F   buphthalmos

9.17.   Which of the following statements are true?

A   in children with ulcerative colitis erythema nodosum is a common skin manifestation

B   secondary syphilitic eruption may mimic pityriasis rosea

C   typical sites affected by psoriasis are elbows and knees

D   patients with chronic atopic eczema may develop cataracts

E   photosensitivity reactions are more severe over body areas not exposed to sunlight

9.18.   In varicella (chickenpox)

A   the rash begins on the trunk

B   the virus can be demonstrated in chickenpox 'crusts'

C   haemorrhagic lesions may occur in patients on steroid therapy

D   lesions are typically in different stages in one anatomical area

E   myocarditis may result

9.19.   In the differential diagnosis of nodular lesions of the ear the following should be considered

A   lepromatous leprosy

B   gout

C   chondrodermatitis helicis nodularis

D   rheumatic fever

E   sarcoidosis

F   lupus vulgaris

9.20.   Pruritus vulvae may be a result of

A   threadworm infestation

B   haemorrhoids

C   epithelioma of the vulva

D   pediculosis pubis

E   lichen sclerosus et atrophicus

F   vaginal infection due to *Trichomonas vaginalis*

PAPER TEN

10.1. Accepted clinical features of psoriasis are

A   ulcerated lesions over buccal mucosa
B   pitting of nails
C   clubbing
D   development of a typical lesion at the site of an operation scar
E   erythematous lesions with silvery scales
F   arthritis

10.2. Cutaneous and renal involvement as a result of the same disease process occurs in

A   alkaptonuria
B   sarcoidosis
C   Henoch–Schönlein purpura
D   gout
E   tuberculosis
F   primary cutaneous amyloidosis

10.3. Skin and gut lesions occur in

A   Peutz–Jeghers syndrome
B   ulcerative colitis
C   Gardner's syndrome
D   acute intermittent porphyria
E   chronic constipation
F   Plummer–Vinson syndrome

10.4. Match the following:

A   Charcot joint
B   histoplasmosis
C   actinomycosis
D   aspergillosis
E   mucormycosis
F   pertussis
1   petechial haemorrhages, periorbital oedema, and hilar lymphadenopathy
2   'sulphur granules', multiple abscesses, and sinuses
3   diabetes mellitus and gangrenous nasal mucosa
4   calcification of spleen and peribronchial lymph nodes
5   'fungus ball' and asthma
6   syringomyelia and tabes dorsalis

10.5. Rheumatoid or rheumatoid-like arthritis can be a feature of

A   lupus erythematosus
B   psoriasis
C   ulcerative colitis
D   acromegaly
E   haemophilia
F   Reiter's syndrome

10.6. Intracranial calcification and cutaneous signs occur in

A   Sturge–Weber syndrome
B   tuberous sclerosis
C   cysticercosis
D   craniopharyngioma
E   toxoplasmosis
F   idiopathic hypoparathyroidism

10.7. Polyarteritis nodosa may present as

A   small haemorrhagic blisters in the skin
B   crops of subcutaneous nodules
C   livedo reticularis
D   Raynaud's phenomenon of late onset
E   pyrexia of unknown origin
F   hypertension
G   abdominal pain

10.8. Disorders that may exhibit both skin lesions and hilar lymphadenopathy include

A   measles
B   molluscum contagiosum
C   infectious mononucleosis
D   sporotrichosis
E   dermatitis herpetiformis
F   varicella

10.9. Skin markers and retarded bone age could be manifestations of

A   adrenogenital syndrome
B   hypopituitarism
C   phenylketonuria
D   Cushing's syndrome
E   juvenile rheumatoid arthritis (Still's disease)
F   hypothyroidism

10.10. Radiology in systemic sclerosis may reveal

A   subperiosteal erosion of the phalanges
B   oesophageal stricture
C   hiatus hernia
D   colonic diverticulae
E   cystic lesions in lung fields
F   dilated air-containing oesophagus

10.11. Diffuse pulmonary fibrosis and specific cutaneous signs are recognised features of

A   neurofibromatosis
B   irradiation of the thorax
C   sarcoidosis
D   psoriasis
E   dermatomyositis

10.12. Hirsutism can be a conspicuous sign in

A   Cushing's syndrome
B   Stein–Leventhal syndrome
C   congenital adrenal hyperplasia
D   arrhenoblastoma
E   Sheehan's syndrome
F   dystrophia myotonica

10.13. Bullous lesions are an expected finding in

A   porphyria cutanea tarda
B   pemphigoid
C   congenital syphilis
D   pityriasis rosea
E   lupus vulgaris
F   scabies
G   erythema multiforme

10.14. Clinical features of dermatomyositis include

A   yellow nails
B   heliotrope erythema over the face
C   periorbital oedema
D   dilated nail fold capillaries
E   calcinosis cutis
F   macroglossia

10.15. Necrobiosis lipoidica diabeticorum

A   occurs more commonly in men
B   characteristic lesions appear on the shins
C   long-standing plaques may ulcerate
D   control of the diabetic state leads to resolution of necrobiosis
E   may precede diabetes mellitus by many years

10.16. Herpes zoster may be induced by

A   previous herpes simplex infection
B   injection of arsenicals
C   Hodgkin's disease
D   lymphatic leukaemia
E   steroid therapy
F   local trauma

10.17. Match the following

A   systemic sclerosis
B   Rothmund–Thomson syndrome
C   scleroedema
D   Takayasu's disease
E   sarcoidosis
F   Werner's syndrome

1   previous streptococcal infection, involvement of hands and feet rare
2   thin pigmented facial skin, absence of radial pulses, increase of blood pressure in lower extremities
3   baldness, grey hair, premature cataracts, sexual underdevelopment
4   lymphadenopathy, cutaneous infiltration of old scars, cor pulmonale
5   Raynaud's phenomenon, malabsorption, calcinosis cutis
6   hyperpigmentation, depigmentation, telangiectasia

10.18. Which of the following contributes to the diagnosis of dermatomyositis?

A   raised serum creatine phosphokinase
B   elevated serum aldolase level
C   radiology showing calcification in muscles
D   presence of antinuclear factor
E   leucopenia
F   increased 24-hour urinary creatine
G   muscle biopsy showing variable degeneration of muscle

10.19. Dermatitis herpetiformis

A   females are affected more frequently than males
B   characteristic eruption consists of grouped vesicles
C   pruritus is usually a predominant symptom
D   bullae when present are intra-epidermal in site
E   jejunal biopsy reveals abnormal mucosa in majority
F   dapsone therapy is effective in controlling skin lesions

10.20. Splinter haemorrhages in nails are a feature of

A   trichinosis
B   lymphatic leukaemia
C   subacute bacterial endocarditis
D   hypertension
E   carcinoid syndrome
F   severe rheumatoid arthritis

ANSWERS

PAPER ONE

1.1. A, B, C, D, and E.

Comment: Several drugs produce an eruption identical with or virtually indistinguishable from lichen planus. Gold and organic arsenicals were amongst the first to be recognised as drugs which produced a lichenoid rash. Arsenic is now considered outdated as a therapeutic measure, but gold appears to have gained in popularity for the treatment of rheumatoid arthritis.

Mepacrine was found to induce a lichenoid eruption as long ago as World War II, when troops who took the drug as an anti-malarial agent developed the typical rash. Chloroquine will also cause a lichenoid eruption and the thiazide diuretics, chlorothiazide and hydrochlorothiazide, are known to have caused a photosensitive lichenoid eruption.

Amiphenazole, a respiratory stimulant, may cause bone marrow depression with long-term usage, but lichenoid eruptions may also be induced.

Methyldopa is an anti-hypertensive agent, the side effects of which include haemolytic anaemia, jaundice, lupus-like syndrome, and a lichenoid eruption.

1.2. A, B, and D.

Comment: The cause of dermatomyositis is not known, but it is associated with carcinoma in adults. The primary tumour is commonly in the lung, breast, or gastro-intestinal tract. In the Chinese, nasopharyngeal carcinoma is the most common underlying malignant disease.

Patients usually exhibit a proximal myopathy, but muscles involved in respiration, in speech, and in swallowing may also be affected, which results in much disability.

Malignancy is not associated with dermatomyositis in childhood.

Of patients with calcinosis, 90% or more are female. The calcinosis usually increases with time and appears to be associated with a good prognosis.

The neoplasm associated with dermatomyositis may precede it, both conditions may appear together, or the dermatomyositis may occur before the neoplasm, as in an estimated 15% of cases.

1.3. A, C, and E.

Comment: The treatment of hyperhidrosis includes topical therapy with aluminium salts, commonly the chlorhydrate or chloride, and iontophoresis, especially for excessive sweating of the hands and feet. Atropine-like drugs help in countering the effects of acetylcholine on sweat glands, but in adequate dosage they produce side effects worse than the hyperhidrosis.

Sympathectomy will cause anhidrosis, but the benefits are only enjoyed for a few years as sweating often returns because of regeneration of sympathetic fibres. Thrombo-angiitis obliterans or Buerger's disease may be helped by sympathectomy in selected cases. Anti-coagulants, corticosteroid therapy, and vasodilators do not help.

Martorell's ulcer is a painful, slow healing ulcer over the lower limbs and occurs predominantly in women over 50 years of age. It has been associated with hypertension – control of this and sympathectomy accelerate healing.

1.4. A – F, B – E, C – A, D – C, E – D, F – B.

1.5. A and E.

Comment: Erythema nodosum commonly occurs over the shins, but lesions may also appear on the thighs and forearms. It usually heals without scarring or atrophy, which helps to differentiate the lesions from those of nodular vasculitis, which may heal with atrophy.

Bilateral hilar lymphadenopathy occurs in infectious diseases in childhood, in Hodgkin's disease, in tuberculosis, and in sarcoidosis, in all of which erythema nodosum may also develop.

Erythema nodosum does not ulcerate.

Arthralgia occurs in over 50% of patients whatever the aetiology. The knee joints are commonly affected and total resolution is the rule.

1.6. A, B, D, and E.

Comment: The pemphigus group of diseases comprises pemphigus vulgaris, pemphigus vegetans, pemphigus foliaceus, and pemphigus erythematosus. All demonstrate serum antibodies against squamous epithelial intercellular spaces. Pemphigus vulgaris is the most common form of pemphigus and, like the other forms, exhibits acantholysis of epidermal cells. This leads to bulla formation, which is situated in the epidermis and therefore ruptures easily. The disease may present as oral ulceration or an isolated scalp lesion and may remain localised for several weeks or months before becoming more widespread.

With systemic corticosteroid therapy the prognosis of pemphigus patients has improved considerably. Prior to corticosteroids 50% died within a year. The mortality rate with present therapy is less than 10% over a 5-year period.

1.7. NONE.

Comment: Ultraviolet light may trigger the onset of SLE or exacerbate the disease. Vitamin C in large doses has helped some patients with miliaria (prickly heat), but there is no evidence that it is a useful therapeutic agent in SLE.

Phenylbutazone is one of many drugs which may induce an SLE-like syndrome. It may also cause blood dyscrasias – agranulocytosis, aplastic anaemia, and thrombocytopenia – after a small dose; in SLE, where thrombocytopenia may occur as part of the disease process, the drug is probably best avoided.

The ESR is raised in some 90% of patients, but may be normal in some throughout the illness so it is not a good guide of disease activity. Anti-malarials are not as useful in SLE as they are in discoid lupus erythematosus; for long-term therapy they may be dangerous.

1.8. A, C, and E.

Comment: Humans are infected with brucellosis by the ingestion of infected milk or other dairy products, or by direct contact with diseased animals.

Specific agglutinins in a titre greater than 1:100 should be regarded as suggestive of infection and when over 1:300 as diagnostic. A positive skin test with Brucella antigen is evidence only of past infection and does not necessarily imply active infection.

Contact with the secretions of an infected animal causes pruritus and weals, which then give rise to a profuse papular eruption. Systemic brucellosis responds well to tetracycline therapy.

1.9. A, B, C, E, and F.

Comment: Facial palsy is a frequent neurological presentation and may occur alone or in association with other cranial nerve palsies.

In sarcoidosis, thymus-derived lymphocytes (T-cells) are depleted, which results in depression of delayed-type hypersensitivity as demonstrated by cutaneous anergy to tuberculin and other antigens.

The Kveim test is positive in 60–75% of active cases. False positive reactions are rare and have occurred in Crohn's disease, brucellosis, and tuberculosis.

Systemic corticosteroid therapy is indicated when hypercalcaemia, but not hypercalciuria, complicates sarcoidosis. Calcium levels may also be lowered by a low calcium diet and oral phosphates.

1.10. A, B, C, D, and E.

Comment: Herpetic keratoconjunctivitis will respond to nucleoside analogues, idoxuridine (IDU), and adenine arabinoside, but ophthalmic preparations of 0.1% IDU in ointment or solution do not appear to alter the course of recurrent herpes labialis, herpes genitalis, or herpetic whitlow. 5% IDU in dimethyl sulphoxide (DMSO) does reduce the duration of lesions in the latter group, but the recurrence rate is not altered significantly. Because the neonatal immune system is poorly developed, herpes simplex in the newborn can spread rapidly and life-threatening meningo-encephalitis and hepatitis may develop. Treatment has included the use of type-specific immunoglobulin, adenine arabinoside intravenously, and, more recently, acycloguanosine.

Gingivostomatitis or vulvovaginitis are usually features of primary herpes simplex that commonly occur in the first 5 years of life. The lesions heal within 2–3 weeks. Eczema herpeticum or Kaposi's varicelliform eruption is an occasional, but potentially life-threatening, complication of eczema, usually of the atopic variety, and results in the development of herpetic lesions over areas involved in atopic eczema, although the lesions may extend to apparently normal skin.

In herpes simplex encephalitis the patient may present with fever, fits, headache, or personality change, or in a coma. Acyclovir, an antiviral agent active *in vitro* against herpes simplex virus (HSV) types I and II, is the treatment of choice. It is most effective if given early. In herpetic keratoconjunctivitis 3% acyclovir ointment is used.

1.11. A, C, E, F, and G.

Comment: Reiter's disease may follow diarrhoeal illness and, in a small percentage of patients, develops after an attack of bacillary dysentery. The disease commonly affects young men and, when venereally acquired, is ushered in by urethritis followed by arthritis and conjunctivitis 10–14 days later. In enteric cases, the diarrhoea is also followed first by urethritis and then by arthritis and conjunctivitis, each developing usually within 10 days of each other.

Keratoderma blennorrhagicum forms in about 8% of venereal cases and only in some 1% of post-dysenteric patients. The feet, both the plantar and dorsal surfaces, the extensor aspects of the legs, and the hands, nails and scalp are commonly involved. Keratoderma is usually self-limiting.

Thrombophlebitis of the deep calf veins may complicate active arthritis of the knee joint.

1.12. A, B, C, D, and F.

Comment: Sunlight is known to exacerbate dermatomyositis, though action spectrum studies have not been described so far.

Porphyria cutanea tarda is frequently diagnosed by the presence of fragile skin over the sun-exposed areas of the body, in particular the backs of the hands.

Pellagra is due to deficiency of niacin. The clinical triad consists of dermatitis, diarrhoea, and dementia. The dermatitic changes are precipitated by the sun and tend to improve in the winter. The lesions are restricted to sun-exposed areas and initially resemble a prolonged sun-burn reaction. When the condition becomes chronic, the skin thickens and may become sclerotic.

Sunlight aggravates rosacea in many patients, but it has also been observed that in one-third of patients exposure to sunlight may improve the condition.

1.13. A, B, C, D, and E.

Comment: Livedo reticularis is a temporary or permanent cyanotic mottling of the skin in a net-like pattern. It may form as a 'secondary' manifestation of diseases, such as polyarteritis nodosa, cryoglobulinaemia, thrombocythaemia, hyperparathyroidism, or tuberculosis.

The lesions in such cases tend to be patchy and asymmetrical. Diffuse arterial disease gives rise to a diffuse mottling of the skin, whereas patchy arterial disease causes patchy mottling.

Livedo reticularis may also occur in rheumatoid arthritis as one manifestation of the arteritic process.

1.14. A, B, C, and D.

Comment: Bleomycin is an antineoplastic drug obtained from *Streptomyces verticillus*, a strain of Actinomycetales. It is used in the treatment of squamous cell carcinomas (other than in the lung), Hodgkin's disease, and embryonal cell carcinoma of the testis. Recognised side effects include pulmonary and skin fibrosis. Patients develop nodules or plaques and occasionally generalised skin induration. The induration occurs commonly on the hands and can result in gangrene of the digits, as seen in scleroderma. The disease is self-limiting and may resolve spontaneously within 2 months of discontinuation of treatment.

Pentazocine injections in drug or alcohol abusers may cause local or generalised cutaneous sclerosis. Induration of the skin may occur within 2 weeks or as late as 3 years after the first injection. Fibrosis of the skin and muscle may be accompanied by ulcers and calcinosis of fat and muscle. Laboratory data are usually negative, except for a high erythrocyte sedimentation rate.

Ingestion of denatured rapeseed oil, sold illegally in Spain, resulted in the outbreak in 1981 of a new clinical syndrome known as the toxic oil syndrome (TOS). The syndrome is ushered in with fever, eosinophilia, pruritus, an erythematous rash, myalgia, arthralgia, dyspnoea, and non-cardiac oedema. The chronic stage of TOS consisted of peripheral neuropathy and skin tightness, simulating scleroderma with several other features, including Raynaud's phenomenon, oesophageal hypomotility, and the development of auto-antibodies. Pulmonary oedema and thrombo-embolic complications were the common causes of death.

A scleroderma-like syndrome has been described in workers involved in the manufacture of PVC. The syndrome consists of Raynaud's phenomenon, sclerodermatous changes in the hands and forearms, and osteolytic and sclerotic bone lesions. It is estimated that some 3% of workers who are exposed develop the disease.

1.15. B, C, D, E, F, and G.

Comment: A photosensitiser is a substance which produces an abnormal reaction in the skin after exposure to light. Photosensitivity may be caused by agents applied to the skin or by drugs administered systemically.

Demeclocycline hydrochloride appears to be the most common photosensitiser in the tetracycline group of drugs, although all tetracyclines have some photosensitising potential. Sulphonamides may photosensitise, and tolbutamide and chlorpropamide, which are chemically related drugs, may also do so. Amongst the phenothiazines, chlorpromazine and promethazine are recognised offenders.

Furocoumarins or psoralens are now widely used in the treatment of psoriasis and other dermatoses, in combination with long-wave ultra violet light (PUVA). The therapy relies on the photosensitising property of psoralen.

Oil of Bergamot, from Bergamot oranges, contains 5-methoxypsoralen, a naturally occurring furocoumarin, and may be found in some perfumes and colognes. A photodermatitis occurs following exposure to sunlight; this is also known as berloque dermatitis.

Halogenated salicylanilides induce a true photoallergic reaction. They have been used as anti-bacterials in soap and one in particular, tetrachlorsalicylanilide, now withdrawn, caused an epidemic of photodermatitis.

1.16. A, B, C, D, and E.

Comment: Morphoea is characterised by sclerosis of the skin. Localised trauma may be the trigger factor in some patients and morphoea can develop as quickly as 18 hours after injury. Pregnancy also appears to exacerbate or provoke morphoea. Frontoparietal lesions that resemble a sabre cut, hence 'en coup de sabre', may involve the skull bones, and the EEG may show dysrhythmia maximal over the affected area. Spina bifida is a common associated abnormality, especially with linear morphoea of the legs, lower abdomen, and buttocks. Abnormalities in the spine have been found on X-ray in almost 50% of patients.

1.17. B, D, E, and F.

Comment: Yaws is a non-venereal, non-congenital, but contagious treponemal disease. *T. pertenue*, the spirochaete responsible, is morphologically indistinguishable from the treponemata of syphilis and pinta.

In the secondary stage of the disease the soles are involved and, to a lesser extent, the palms. A plantar keratoderma develops, which fissures and is extremely painful. The patient adopts a peculiar gait to avoid pain on walking and this has provided the descriptive term 'crab yaws'. Periostitis and osteitis occur in the late or tertiary stage. The overlying skin may be invaded and ulcerate. Serological tests for syphilis are positive in both yaws and pinta.

1.18. A, B, C and F.

Comment: Infectious mononucleosis is caused by a herpes virus, usually referred to as the Epstein–Barr virus. A sore throat commonly develops a few days prior to the onset of the illness and multiple petechiae at the junction of the hard and soft palates are a distinctive feature.

The liver is often involved, although in practice jaundice is uncommon. Thrombocytopenic purpura also occurs, but again is a rare complication. The incidence of a rash is vastly increased by the administration of Ampicillin and usually occurs within 10 days of treatment.

1.19. B, C, and E.

Comment: Chronic venous ulceration is often associated with previous deep-vein thrombosis. Ante-natal and post-partum thrombosis accounts for a significant number of cases. Trauma, thrombophlebitis, and therapy such as varicose vein treatment with sclerosants or abdominal operations, are other recognised causes. Subcutaneous calcification occurs in 10% of patients with chronic venous stasis and it may be responsible for the non-healing of an ulcer. Serum calcium and phosphorus are normal.

Periostitis is commonly seen under a chronic ulcer. Lymphoedema is another complication of the post-thrombotic leg. The superficial lymphatics are absent under and around ulcers, and if there is pre-existing dysfunction of the lymphatic system, cellulitis tends to occur fairly commonly. Malignant change in a venous ulcer is very rare indeed.

1.20. A, B, D, and E.

Comment: The typical lesions of arteritis in rheumatoid arthritis are painless, periungual infarcts. They are usually transitory and may be missed.

There appears to be a greater incidence of arteritis in patients who receive systemic corticosteroid therapy, and lesions may form with cessation of the therapy or a change in the dose of steroids.

Leg ulcers may also form as a result of arteritis or may simply be gravitational. Arteritic ulcers are common in men, particularly those with subcutaneous nodules, and are typically deep and punched-out. Leg ulcers also occur in Felty's syndrome, in which arthritis is associated with splenomegaly and leucopenia.

Subcutaneous nodules occur in some 20% of patients with rheumatoid arthritis. The commonest site is the ulnar border of the forearm. These usually signify severe rheumatoid arthritis, although they may occasionally precede the disease by many years or be associated with mild arthritis.

PAPER ONE

FURTHER READING

Browne, S.G. (1976), Treponemal depigmentation with special reference to yaws, *South African Medical Journal*, **50**, 442.

Buchanan, T.M., Faber, L.C., and Feldman, R.A. (1974), Brucellosis in the United States, 1960–1972. An abattoir-associated disease. Part 1. Clinical features and therapy, *Medicine*, **53**, 403.

Bywaters, E.G.L. and Scott, J.T. (1963), The natural history of vascular lesions in rheumatoid arthritis, *Journal of Chronic Diseases*, **16**, 905.

Caird, F.I. and Holt, P.R. (1958), The enanthem of glandular fever, *British Medical Journal*, **1**, 85.

Callen, J.P., Hyla, J.F., Bole, G.G., *et al.* (1980), The relationship of dermatomyositis and polymyositis to internal malignancy, *Archives of Dermatology*, **116**, 295.

Carlisle, J.W. and Good, R.A. (1959), Dermatomyositis in childhood: report of studies on several cases and review of the literature, *Lancet*, **79**, 266.

Chorzelski, T.P., von Weiss, J.V., and Lever, W.F. (1966), Clinical significance of autoantibodies in pemphigus, *Archives of Dermatology*, **93**, 570.

Csonka, G. (1966), Thrombophlebitis in Reiter's syndrome, *British Journal of Venereal Diseases*, **42**, 93.

Epstein, J.H., Tuffanelli, D., and Dubois, E.L. (1965), Light sensitivity and lupus erythematosus, *Archives of Dermatology*, **91**, 483.

Greenhaigh, R.M., Rosengarten, D.S., and Martin, P. (1971), Role of sympathectomy for hyperhidrosis, *British Medical Journal*, **1**, 332.

Harber, L.C. and Baer, R.L. (1972), Pathogenic mechanisms of drug-induced photosensitivity, *Journal of Investigative Dermatology*, **58**, 327.

Knight, V. and Noall, N.W. (1976), Recurrent herpes, *New England Journal of Medicine*, **294**, 337.

Lippman, H.I. and Goldin, R.R. (1960), Subcutaneous ossification of the legs in chronic venous insufficiency, *Radiology*, **74**, 279.

Logan, R.A. and Griffiths, W.A.D. (1989), Climatic factors and rosacea, in *Acne and Related Disorders*, R. Marks and G. Plewig (Eds), Martin Dunitz, London, p. 311.

Montgomery, M.M., Poske, R.M., Barton, E.M., *et al.*, (1959), The mucocutaneous lesions of Reiter's syndrome, *Annals of Internal Medicine*, **51**, 99.

Palestine, R.F. and Rogers, R.S., III (1982), Diagnosis and treatment of mycetoma, *Journal of the American Academy of Dermatology*, **6**, 107.

Rimington, C., Magnus, I.A., Ryan, E., *et al.* (1967), Porphyria and photosensitivity, *Quarterly Journal of Medicine*, **36**, 29.

Rosenberg, F.R., Sanders, S., and Nelson, C.T. (1976), Pemphigus: a 20 year review of 107 patients treated with corticosteroids, *Archives of Dermatology*, **112**, 962.

Willcox, R.R. (1964), *Textbook of Venereal Diseases and Treponematoses*, C. C. Thomas, Springfield, Illinois.

PAPER TWO

2.1. A, B, C, D, E, F, and G.

Comment: Many different provocative factors are recognised for erythema multiforme. The commonest association is with a preceding herpes simplex or Mycoplasma infection. Vaccinia, pregnancy, and a variety of drugs, which include phenylbutazone, barbiturates, penicillin, aspirin, and sulphonamides, are other recognized causes.

2.2. A, B, C, D, E, F, and G.

Comment: Palmar erythema, spider angiomata, white nail beds, diffuse pigmentation, loss of axillary and pubic hair, and gynaecomastia are all well-described signs of hepatic failure. None of these signs should be considered specific for liver disease. Hyperoestrogenism is thought to be responsible for the gynaecomastia and spider naevi, whilst hypo-albuminaemia underlies the development of some white nails. If there is an obstructive element, xanthomata may occur.

2.3. A, B, C, and E.

Comment: Premature greying is notably increased in a number of diseases associated with organ-specific auto-antibodies. In thyrotoxicosis and other thyroid disorders, and in pernicious anaemia, there is a significantly increased incidence of premature greying.

In dystrophia myotonica, male pattern alopecia is a feature, but premature greying may precede or accompany the muscle disease. In progeria the process of ageing is accelerated and hair reflects this by becoming sparse and prematurely grey. In tuberous sclerosis a strand or mesh of white hairs (poliosis) has been found in 60% of cases.

2.4. B, C, D, and E.

Comment: Macroglossia refers to an inappropriately enlarged tongue, relative to the size of the mouth and jaws. In cretinism and myxoedema, the tongue can be symmetrically enlarged. Oedematous macroglossia may occur as part of angioneurotic oedema or as a result of a wasp or bee sting on the tongue itself.

In primary amyloidosis enlargement of the tongue occurs in 30–40% of patients. Median rhomboid glossitis presents as loss of papillae in the mid-line of the tongue. The affected area is usually seen as a smooth plaque. The condition is not pre-malignant and does not require treatment. In some patients *Candida albicans* has been cultured and the glossitis has cleared with appropriate anti-Candida therapy.

2.5. A, B, C, D, and E.

Comment: Primary infection with *Herpesvirus hominis* gives rise to herpetic gingivostomatitis, which is the commonest cause of stomatitis in 1–6-year-old children. A few vesicles on the oral mucosa often accompany the lesions of varicella on the body, but usually do not prove troublesome. Oral lesions may occur in herpes zoster when the second or third division of the trigeminal nerve is involved. Grouped vesicles develop on the buccal mucosa, tongue, palate, and gingiva.

Hand, foot, and mouth disease presents with stomatitis, especially in children. Caused by Coxsackie viruses type A16, A10, and A5, the infection occurs in small outbreaks, but spreads rapidly within closed communities. Superficial vesicles appear in the mouth and on the hands and feet, and generally heal within a week.

Herpangina, also caused by viruses of Coxsackie group A, is predominantly a disease of children. It is characterised by a sore throat, pyrexia, and dysphagia. Small discrete vesicles, each surrounded by a band of erythema, may be seen over the palate, fauces, and pharynx.

2.6. B, D, E, F, and G.

Comment: Waardenburg's syndrome includes perceptive deafness, associated with a white forelock and premature greying of the hair, which may occur in the third decade.

The Chediak–Higashi syndrome is inherited as an autosomal recessive gene. There is hypopigmentation of the skin, hair, and eyes. Patients show an increased susceptibility to infection, and intractable skin and respiratory infections commonly result in death before the age of 10 years.

Incontinentia pigmenti is inherited as an X-linked dominant trait, though spontaneous mutations do occur. The disease is usually lethal in males and presents with tense blisters at birth in female infants. The pigmentation is characteristic, being described as 'splashed' or resembling 'Chinese lettering', and persists for many years, but has usually faded by the second or third decade.

Pigmentation in adults with Gaucher's disease may be seen as prominent patches on the face, neck, and hands, or as a symmetrical pigmentation of the lower legs.

2.7. A, B, and C.

Comment: Erythroderma (literally 'red skin') is a secondary process and results from the generalisation of a pre-existing skin disease, usually eczema or psoriasis. It may occasionally be a manifestation of a drug hypersensitivity and rarely a sign of a systemic disease.

In long-standing or recurrent erythroderma, lymphadenopathy is a common finding, but a lymph node biopsy is seldom useful in differentiating the various causes of erythroderma.

The regulation of temperature is usually markedly abnormal and hypothermia is a serious risk. An increase in body temperature leads to an increase in heat loss. The increased blood flow through the skin may result, in turn, in a high-output cardiac failure.

2.8. A, B, C, D, and E.

Comment: Darier's disease is inherited as an autosomal dominant trait. The typical skin lesions are firm greasy papules, which occur as grouped lesions, commonly over the scalp, face, flexures, and trunk. Severely affected individuals are often of small stature and low intelligence.

Hartnup disease is characterised by a pellagrous eruption associated with neurological manifestations, the commonest being cerebellar ataxia. Less commonly there are psychological disturbances, such as depression and hallucinations, and mental retardation may be an associated feature.

2.9. A, B, C, D, and F.

Comment: Erythema nodosum is an early feature of sarcoidosis and is usually associated with bilateral hilar lymphadenopathy (Stage 1) and a good prognosis.

Lupus pernio commonly affects young or middle-aged women and is usually apparent on the nose, cheeks, ears, or hands. Nasal involvement may occur and be severe enough to cause difficulty in breathing. Erosion of the nasal bones is a recognised complication. Lupus pernio occurs in the chronic stage of sarcoid and is associated with fusiform swelling of the fingers in 10–20% of patients.

Sarcoidosis of the scalp usually results in scarring alopecia.

2.10. C and D.

Comment: Bilharziasis, or visceral schistosomiasis, is caused by the human blood flukes *Schistosoma mansoni, S. japonicum,* and *S. haematobium.* Eggs excreted in faeces or urine develop into miracidia on contact with water. After further development in aquatic snails, free-swimming cercariae are released, which can penetrate human skin to cause bilharziasis.

African trypanosomiasis is transmitted by tsetse flies, whilst American trypanosomiasis is transmitted by winged bugs.

Kala-azar (literally black fever), or visceral leishmaniasis, is caused by a protozoon, *Leishmania donovani,* transmitted by a Phlebotomus sandfly.

Cysticercosis results from ingestion of the larva, *Cysticercus cellulosae,* of the adult *Taenia solium* or pork tapeworm. These may be transmitted in contaminated food or water or from hands which have been inadequately cleaned.

2.11. A, B, D, E, and F.

Comment: Erythema over the 'butterfly area' of the face is not specific to lupus erythematosus and occurs in a variety of conditions, which include rosacea, carcinoid, and dermatomyositis.

Suffusion of the face may be seen in polycythaemia rubra vera and superior vena caval obstruction. In practice, rosacea is probably the commonest cause of a malar erythema and is differentiated from the SLE rash by the absence of pustules in the latter.

Although seborrhoeic dermatitis may present as areas of erythema in the rosaceous area, it is usually associated with scaling, which is an important differentiating sign.

As the name implies, patients with solar urticaria develop urticaria on exposure to sunlight or artificial radiation. Many patients develop lesions only when they expose skin that is normally shielded from light by clothing, and skin that is routinely exposed, such as on the face, may be unaffected.

2.12. A, B, C, D, E, F, G, and H.

Comment: The hypopituitary dwarf is usually bald. In Sheehan's syndrome, the scalp hair becomes thin, and pubic and axillary hair are also lost.

Diffuse loss of scalp hair is frequent in hypothyroidism. Sparsity of eyebrows may be obvious, but regrowth to a variable degree occurs when the patient is euthyroid again.

In hyperthyroidism diffuse alopecia develops in 40–50% of cases, but it is also reversible. Some patients with thyrotoxicosis that has been treated with anti-thyroid agents develop diffuse alopecia.

In hypoparathyroidism the scalp hair is easily shed with slight trauma and the alopecia appears patchy.

Excessive consumption of vitamin A results in a slowly progressive thinning of scalp hair, eyebrows, and eyelashes. Loss of weight, lethargy, anaemia, and bone pain are frequent symptoms; they develop after doses in excess of 50 000 units daily have been taken for many months.

In homocystinuria, an inborn error in the metabolic pathway of methionine, the hair is sparse, fine, and fair. Affected children are mentally retarded and show a variety of skeletal defects.

2.13. A, B, C, D, and F.

Comment: In diabetes and arteriosclerosis, the reduced arterial supply predisposes to ulcer formation.

Indolent ulcers of the skin are a feature of sickle-cell anaemia, hereditary spherocytosis, and other haemolytic anaemias.

Embolism or thrombosis of the anterior tibial artery as a result of unaccustomed exertion, polyarteritis nodosa, or cardiac disease causes severe pain in the anterior tibial area. Swelling and pain herald ischaemic necrosis and immediate surgery is required.

In Still's disease (juvenile rheumatoid arthritis) multiple painful ulcers may occur on the legs and feet; these are difficult to heal, though low molecular weight dextran and sympathectomy are of some help.

Barbiturate poisoning may result in a few tense, thick-walled bullae, usually on the lower limbs, but leg ulceration is not a recognised feature.

2.14. A, B, D, E, F, and G.

Comment: Many diseases cause an increase in gammaglobulin . Almost all infections will do so, although it may not be sufficient to show an abnormality on paper electrophoresis. Chronic infections characteristically show an increase, especially tuberculosis.

Sjögren's syndrome and lupus erythematosus often result in considerably raised values.

Sarcoidosis and lymphogranuloma venereum are other well-described aetiologies.

Gammaglobulin is frequently increased in Hodgkin's disease, malignant lymphoma, and chronic lymphatic leukaemia.

Another category for gammaglobulinaemia is the group of liver diseases. In cirrhosis there is typically a marked increase, though in some 10% of patients there may be no gamma elevation. In obstructive jaundice, one often sees an increase in alpha-2, beta, and gammaglobulin to a varying degree.

In the nephrotic syndrome there is secondary hypogammaglobulinaemia.

2.15. A, B, C, D, and E.

Comment: Hypertrichosis of exposed skin is a common feature of erythropoietic porphyria, and is also seen in the more common erythropoietic protoporphyria. The hypertrichosis is best seen on the temples, forehead, and cheeks, though it may also occur on other light-exposed areas.

In Hurler's syndrome, hypertrichosis is usually present from infancy or early childhood. The eyebrows are often bushy and increased hair growth may also be apparent on the trunk and limbs.

Coarse hair is often present over the plaques of pretibial myxoedema.

An increased growth of fine, downy hair, usually widespread on the body, is described in approximately 20% of patients with anorexia nervosa.

2.16. A, B, C, D, E, and F.

Comment: In sickle-cell disease, chronic leg ulcers that overlie the malleoli tend to occur at puberty or later. Hyposthenuria is the most common evidence of renal dysfunction. Renal infarcts or papillary necrosis can cause haematuria and recurrent infarction may lead to progressive renal insufficiency. Occasionally, renal vein thrombosis occurs, and may result in the nephrotic syndrome.

In hereditary haemorrhagic telangiectasia, the small flattened telangiectases on the skin may be associated with lesions in the respiratory and genito-urinary systems, though they are commonest in the gastro-intestinal tract.

2.17. B, C, D, E, and F.

Comment: Onycholysis is a painless separation of the nail from its bed. The separated area appears pale clinically because of the loss of light reflection from the nail bed. There are many causes of onycholysis, of which fungal infection, psoriasis, and dermatitis are common. Minor trauma is also a common cause, particularly so in certain occupations.

Impaired peripheral circulation (Raynaud's disease), myxoedema, and thyrotoxicosis may also induce onycholysis.

2.18. B, C, D, E, and F.

Comment: In thyrotoxicosis there is increased sweating and the sodium content of the sweat is reduced. Overt sweating usually develops with mild exertion. In 10–15% of patients with autoimmune endocrine disorders, for example Hashimoto's thyroiditis or Graves' disease, there is vitiligo.

Hyperpigmentation is of the Addisonian type and thought to be due to increased ACTH production, because thyroxine results in an increased breakdown of cortisol.

Clubbing of the fingers and toes associated with periosteal new bone formation of the phalanges – thyroid acropachy – is frequently associated with thyrotoxicosis.

Pretibial myxoedema presents as a localised oedematous and thickened pretibial plaque, usually associated with raised levels of long-acting thyroid stimulator (LATS) in the serum. Occasionally, the pretibial patches do not become apparent until after anti-thyroid treatment has been commenced.

2.19. B, C, and D.

Comment: In arterial insufficiency of the lower limbs, the skin becomes thin and dry, or shiny and cyanotic. The hair over the limbs lessens and may be lost from the dorsa of the foot and toes. The nails thicken and become dystrophic.

Intermittent claudication is the classic symptom of arteriosclerosis. There may also be rest pain, especially at night, coldness or paresthesia due to ischaemic neuropathy and increased sensitivity to cold.

The peripheral pulses are usually grossly impaired or absent.

Arterial ulcers are classically painful, punched-out, and with well-defined edges. They are always slow to heal.

2.20. A, C, D, E, and F.

Comment: Diabetes has been reported with all forms of hepatic porphyria and is frequently found in porphyria cutanea tarda.

In total lipo-atrophy (Lawrence–Seip syndrome) diabetes mellitus develops in association with loss of subcutaneous and visceral fat. Other features of the syndrome include hepatomegaly and increased bone growth. In partial lipo-atrophy diabetes mellitus develops in a third of the patients.

Haemochromatosis, which is ten times more common in men, is characterised by a slate-grey/brown pigmentation of the skin, cirrhosis, and hypogonadism. Diabetes occurs in 80% of patients.

PAPER TWO

FURTHER READING

Bleehen, S. (1969), Systemic sarcoidosis with scalp involvement, *Proceedings of the Royal Society of Medicine*, **62**, 348.

Borrie, P. (1953), Rosacea with special reference to its ocular manifestations, *British Journal of Dermatology*, **65**, 458.

Bridges, J.M., Gibson, J.B., Loughbridge, L.W., *et al.* (1975), Carcinoid syndrome with pellagrous dermatitis, *British Journal of Surgery*, **45**, 117.

Brettle, R.P., Gray, J.A., Sangster, G., *et al.* (1982), The mucocutaneous syndromes – erythema multiforme, Stevens–Johnson and ectodermis pluriorificialis, *Journal of Infection*, **4**, 149.

Carson, N.A., Dent, C.E., Field, C.M., *et al.* (1965), Homocystinuria: clinical and pathological review of ten cases, *Journal of Paediatrics*, **66**, 565.

Chevrant-Breton, J., Simon, B., Bourel, M., *et al.* (1977), Cutaneous manifestations of idiopathic haemochromatosis. Study of 100 cases, *Archives of Dermatology*, **113**, 161.

Cunliffe, W.J., Hall, R., Newell, D.J., *et al.* (1968), Vitiligo, thyroid disease and autoimmunity, *British Journal of Dermatology*, **80**, 135.

Eckert, J., Church, R.E., Ebling, F.J., *et al.* (1967), Hair loss in women, *British Journal of Dermatology*, **79**, 543.

Ferriman, D. and Gallwey, J.D. (1961), Clinical assessment of body hair growth in women, *Journal of Clinical Endocrinology and Metabolism*, **21**, 1440.

Higgins, P.G. and Warin, R.P. (1967), Hand, foot and mouth disease: a clinically recognizable virus infection seen mainly in children, *Clinical Paediatrics*, **6**, 373.

Lerner, A.B. (1971), On the etiology of vitiligo and gray hair, *American Journal of Medicine*, **51**, 141.

Lewin, K., DeWit, S., and Ferrington, R.A. (1972), Pathology of the fingernail in psoriasis, *British Journal of Dermatology*, **86**, 555.

Lynch, P.J., Maize, J.C., and Sisson, J.C. (1973), Pretibial myxoedema and nonthyrotoxic thyroid disease, *Archives of Dermatology*, **107**, 107.

Menendez, C.V. (1967), *Ulcers of the Leg. Cause and Treatment*, C. C. Thomas, Springfield, Illinois.

Nickel, W.R. and Reed, W.B. (1962), Tuberous sclerosis. Special reference to the microscopic alterations in the cutaneous hamartomas, *Archives of Dermatology*, **85**, 209.

Sarkany, I. (1969), The skin lesions associated with liver disease, *Progress in Dermatology*, **4**, 1.

Shelley, W.B. (1967), Herpes simplex virus as a cause of erythema multiforme, *Journal of the American Medical Association*, **201**, 153.

Shuster, S. and Marks, J. (1970), *Systemic Effects of Skin Disease*, Heinemann, London.

Terry, R. (1954), White nails in hepatic cirrhosis, *Lancet*, **i**, 757.

Windhorst, D.B., Zelickson, A.S., and Good, R.A. (1968), A human pigmentary dilution based on a heritable subcellular structural defect, the Chediak–Higashi syndrome, *Journal of Investigative Dermatology*, **50**, 9.

PAPER THREE

3.1. A, B, C, D, and E.

Comment: In acute pancreatitis a livedo reticularis may be seen over the abdomen and upper thighs. Also, spread of haemorrhage from the tail of the pancreas along the falciform ligament leads to bruising around the umbilicus (Cullen's sign). This sign may also be seen, for similar reasons, with a perforated duodenal ulcer or in ectopic pregnancy.

Pancreatic disease may be associated with a syndrome consisting of subcutaneous nodules and synovitis of the small or medium sized joints. The nodules usually heal without a depressed scar, but can occasionally ulcerate.

Thrombophlebitis migrans may be due to malignancy; when so pancreatic cancer is found in approximately three out of ten patients.

3.2. B and C.

Comment: In serum sickness, the prototypic form of hypersensitivity, vasculitis is now rarely seen in its classic form, since horse serum is injected into humans only as snake anti-venom. Reactions of the serum sickness type that occur with various drugs, particularly penicillin, are more commonly encountered. Clinical manifestations begin 7–10 days following administration of the drug, with the abrupt onset of fever and arthralgias, followed by headache, abdominal pain, paresthesiae, and glomerulo-nephritis. Urticaria rather than purpura is the usual skin manifestation.

Polyarteritis nodosa may involve virtually any organ system, though it frequently affects the renal and visceral vasculature. Cutaneous lesions may occur in up to 50% of patients and include painful nodules, palpable purpura, or urticaria. Fever, arthralgias, and myalgias frequently accompany the acute phase of the disease.

Fever is not a feature of scurvy.

Takayasu's disease is a rare form of vasculitis that primarily affects medium-to-large arteries, particularly the aortic arch and its branches. It has no cutaneous manifestations.

Temporal arteritis, also called giant cell arteritis, presents commonly with headache, scalp tenderness, and visual impairment. Skin lesions can occur in the form of necrosis or alteration of the skin that overlies the involved artery.

3.3. B, C, D, and F.

Comment: In scabies the mite favours certain areas of the skin, which include the wrist, hands, feet, and genitalia. It is hardly ever, if at all, found on the head or neck.

Erysipelas, a skin infection usually caused by streptococci of group A, frequently occurs over the face and scalp both in children and adults.

Buerger's disease, or thromboangiitis obliterans, affects small and medium sized arteries of the extremities and is common in young males. Most patients are smokers and therapy includes strict abstinence from tobacco.

3.4. A, B, C, E, and F.

Comment: The vast majority of women show a premenstrual exacerbation of acne vulgaris. Many other existing dermatoses become more active, including rosacea, lupus erythematosus, and various forms of eczema.

Anogenital pruritus may become acute premenstrually, but often abates somewhat during menstruation. In some unfortunate women herpes simplex develops regularly during the premenstrual phase and this may present as herpes labialis or the less common herpes genitalis.

3.5. A, C, E, and F.

Comment: The pathogenesis of pyoderma gangrenosum still remains unclear. It is frequently associated with underlying systemic disease, but in a significant number of patients no abnormality is demonstrated.

Pyoderma gangrenosum occurs in patients with leukaemia and, in some, may precede it. The majority of cases described have been associated with acute or chronic myeloid leukaemia.

A recent study found that ulcerative colitis is complicated by pyoderma gangrenosum in some 5% of patients.

Pyoderma gangrenosum may also occur in Crohn's disease and in one study there were six cases in 498 patients with regional enteritis.

3.6. B, C, D, E, and F.

Comment: Ataxia telangiectasia inherited as an autosomal recessive trait is a syndrome characterised by progressive cerebellar ataxia, recurrent chest infections, and telangiectases on the conjunctivae, face, and limbs.

The triad of telangiectasia, erythema, and pustules over the face help to make the diagnosis of rosacea, which is thought to result from prolonged vasodilatation.

Atrophy of skin results in telangiectasia and is recognised as a side effect of topical steroids when used in excess for prolonged periods.

Scurvy, caused by a deficiency of vitamin C in the diet, results in easy bruising with haematoma formation and petechial haemorrhages, especially on the legs.

3.7. A, B, C, D, and E.

Comment: Staphylococcal lesions are more common in diabetics than in non-diabetics. They usually present as carbuncles, boils, or styes.

Pruritus in diabetes is usually localised rather than generalised, and often presents in the genitocrural areas as a dermatophyte or monilial infection.

In untreated diabetes small yellow papules may erupt (eruptive xanthomas) over the trunk and limbs, with a propensity for the elbows, knees, and buttocks. The fasting serum usually shows considerable triglyceridaemia.

Rubeosis refers to a red facies and is believed to be caused by diabetic micro-angiopathy.

3.8. B, C, D, and E.

Comment: Talc granuloma of the umbilicus occurs in infants and very young children. The talc crystals are recognised by their doubly refractile property.

Pyogenic granuloma, a misnomer as it is neither due to infection nor a granuloma on histology, may also occur in the umbilicus. It bleeds readily with trauma and is treated with curettage and cautery under local anaesthetic.

A patent urachus duct is rare, but forms when the umbilical opening is lined by skin or protruding mucous membrane.

3.9. A, B, D, and E.

Comment: Angiomatous or cavernous naevi occur in the first month of life in 90% of cases. At least 90% undergo spontaneous resolution, which is usually complete by the age of 10 years. Ulceration occurs in a minority and is commonest in naevi in the napkin area.

Haemangiomatous involvement of a bone may cause extensive osteolysis and fibrous replacement.

Angiomatous naevi may be associated with thrombocytopenic purpura, the so-called Kasabach–Merritt syndrome. In this situation, prednisolone is the treatment of choice and is given for approximately 3 weeks. Regression of the naevus usually occurs within 2 weeks.

The von Hippel–Lindau syndrome consists of angiomas of skin with angiomatosis of the retina and cerebellum or medulla. Hypernephromas have been reported in 20% of affected patients.

3.10. A, B, C, E, and F.

Comment: Patients with hypocalcaemia show widespread xeroderma and dry scaly skin.

Body hair is generally reduced, with diminution of scalp hair, eyelashes, and eyebrows, and some loss of axillary and pubic hair.

The nails break easily and are often secondarily infected with Candida.

An uncommon manifestation of hypocalcaemia is 'impetigo herpetiformis' – so-called as it presents with grouped pustules on an erythematous base. The skin changes, apart from impetigo herpetiformis, result from chronic hypocalcaemia and respond to calcium replacement therapy.

3.11. A, B, C, D, and E.

Comment: Bone marrow transplantation is frequently used for the treatment of certain leukaemias, aplastic anaemia, and some immunodeficiency diseases. Graft-versus-host disease (GVHD) can develop 10–40 days after transplantation and is characterised by a morbilliform eruption, hepatitis, diarrhoea, and lymphocytopenia.

Other cutaneous features are purpura, hyperpigmentation, and toxic epidermal necrolysis.

Patients who survive 3–4 months may develop chronic GVHD. This syndrome consists of Sjögren's syndrome (keratoconjunctivitis sicca), lichen-planus-like lesions that affect the skin and oral mucosa, cholestatic liver disease, and sclerodermatous skin lesions. Raynaud's phenomenon does not usually occur.

3.12. A, C, D, and E.

Comment: Candidiasis is extremely common in the anogenital areas and may present as a balanitis, vulvovaginitis, or a perianal or scrotal candidiasis. It is often found in pregnancy and, in untreated diabetics, it may be the presenting feature.

Keratoderma blenorrhagica, as part of Reiter's disease, usually occurs after the onset of arthritis and conjunctivitis. The soles of the feet are almost always involved, but the hands and scalp are also common sites.

Pediculosis may involve the scalp, the body, and the genitocrural area. In the hirsute male the infection may be widespread, and in females it may present as intense pruritus vulvae.

Erythrasma occurs commonly in the groin and in the axillae. As the infection is asymptomatic it is often overlooked, but it may be visualised with Wood's lighr, under which the patches fluoresce a distinctive salmon-pink colour.

Hidradenitis suppurativa is a chronic infection of the apocrine sweat glands. Typically, the lesions affect the axillae and the anogenital area. Men are more commonly affected with genitocrural hidradenitis and the majority of these also show acne.

3.13. A, C, D, and E.

Comment: In primary amyloidosis the tongue is enlarged and yellowish nodules may form along its margin.

In diabetes mellitus periodontal disease is common, especially in children. Gingivitis is frequently seen and a periodontal abscess may form.

In Hand–Schüller–Christian disease loosening of teeth is an early manifestation. When the disease involves the gingivae the teeth may be shed. The maxilla and mandible may also be infiltrated.

Lipoid proteinosis is a rare condition characterised by deposition of hyaline material in the skin and mucous membranes. It usually presents in infancy with hoarseness and, later, ulceration of the oral mucosa may occur.

3.14. A, B, C, D, E, F, and G.

Comment: It is estimated that some 10–20 million people in the world suffer from leprosy. A high proportion of leprosy is either transmitted by short direct contact with bacteriologically positive patients or acquired via vectors such as flies, mosquitos, or bedbugs. Patients with lepromatous leprosy are considered to show little or no resistance to *mycobacterium leprae* because of a defect in their cell-mediated immunity that prevents macrophages from killing the parasite.

In untreated leprosy a leonine facies develops and the nose becomes misshapen to produce a saddle nose deformity.

Ulceration of the legs occurs and testicular atrophy causes sterility, impotence, and gynaecomastia.

The only cranial nerves that may suffer damage are those with a course outside the skull; these are the first (olfactory), fifth (trigeminal), and the seventh (facial) nerves.

3.15. A, C, D, and E.

Comment: In oculocutaneous albinism the basic defect is an inability to synthesise melanin because of a defect in the tyrosinase system. This lack of melanin predisposes the skin of these patients to severe actinic damage and premature cutaneous cancer, which are evident usually before 30 years of age.

There are no cutaneous manifestations in acute intermittent porphyria.

Phenylketonuria is also associated with a decreased pigmentation of the skin, the cause being absence or impaired synthesis of the enzyme phenylalanine hydroxylase, which converts phenylalanine into tyrosine. Patients are more susceptible to acute phototoxic injury, although so far it has not been shown that there is a significant increase in skin cancer.

In vitiligo melanocytes are destroyed. The vitiliginous areas become prone to sunburn, although skin cancers are rare, except in vitiligo which is total (universal vitiligo), where chronic sun damage may induce neoplasia.

The Chediak–Higashi syndrome is inherited as an autosomal recessive trait and is characterised by pale skin and a decrease in uveal pigment. These patients therefore sunburn easily and also exhibit nystagmus and photophobia. They are also unusually susceptible to infection, thought to be due to abnormal leucocyte chemotaxis and reduced bacterial killing.

3.16. B, C, D, and F.

Comment: Dithranol, a tar derivative, stains the skin a variable shade of brown, depending on the concentration used.

Pinta, a treponematosis caused by *Treponema carateum*, affects only the skin. It produces depigmented lesions in the late phases of the disease, which may occur over any part of the body, but are frequent over bony prominences, such as the elbows, knees, wrists, and back of the hands.

In tuberculoid leprosy the typical lesion is an erythematous plaque with a hypopigmented centre. Occasionally, a hypopigmented macule forms, particularly in dark skin. The lesions are usually anaesthetic, anhidrotic, and hairless.

Pityriasis alba is an eczema that occurs commonly in children and may present as hypopigmented patches, especially over the face. If very conspicuous it may be mistaken for vitiligo, but the fine scaling and distribution of pityriasis alba helps in differentiation.

3.17. A, B, C, and E.

Comment: The most dreaded complication of a pigmented naevus is its transformation into a malignant melanoma. The risk is greater if an individual has multiple pigmented naevi or if a large naevus has been present from birth. Otherwise, malignant change is rare before puberty.

A sudden increase in the size of a naevus, an uneven surface pigmentation, or pruritus in a naevus are indicators of activity and demand immediate excision of the lesion and histological examination.

Ulceration and bleeding in a naevus are often late signs of a malignant melanoma that has already developed.

3.18. A, B, C, E, F, and G.

Comment: Erythema nodosum is a nodular erythematous eruption which occurs commonly over the shins. It is at least three times more common in women and most cases occur between the ages of 20 and 45 years.

It is generally an early manifestation of sarcoidosis, which is thought to be the commonest cause in Scandinavia.

Tuberculosis, though not now common in the USA and Europe, is still very common in the Third World and should always be excluded.

Streptococcal infections remain an important cause and are often responsible for recurrent attacks of erythema nodosum.

Cat scratch fever is a well-described cause and Yersinia infections have been implicated commonly in France and Finland.

In Behçet's disease nodular lesions occur as a result of thrombosis rather than a primary inflammation of the vessel walls.

3.19. B, C, D, E, F, and G.

Comment: In Darier's disease lesions of the mucous membranes are uncommon, but oral papules may occur, as may gum hypertrophy. Confluence of the papules may resemble patches of leucoplakia.

In bullous pemphigoid blisters in the mouth occur in some 20% of patients and usually late in the disease.

In bullous erythema multiforme or the Stevens–Johnson syndrome oral lesions are severe and invariably present.

The presence of bullae, occasionally haemorrhagic, is an essential feature of benign mucous membrane pemphigoid, in which eye lesions also occur.

In dermatitis herpetiformis oral lesions are uncommon and mild. When present, they are small, grouped, and vesicular, and may be painful after rupture.

In pemphigus vulgaris oral blisters are the presenting feature in the vast majority of patients. They result in intensely painful ulcerated areas and can occur anywhere in the mouth.

3.20. A, C, D, E, and F.

Comment: Contact dermatitis may occur from hypersensitivity to shoes and stockings, and occasionally even from topical therapy. Dermatitis from nylon stockings is caused by an allergy to azodyes, while shoe dermatitis may be caused by a reaction against leather, rubber, or dyes.

Psoriasis may occur on the palms and soles as typical scaly patches, with a silvery scale, or as a pustulosis. Occasionally, it may resemble eczema.

Tinea pedis, or foot ringworm, is commonly caused by one of three dermatophyte fungal species – *Trichophyton rubrum*, *T. interdigitale*, and *Epidermophyton floccosum*.

Cutaneous larva migrans is typified by lesions which 'creep or migrate' and is caused by parasites that move in the skin. *Ancylostoma braziliense* (hookworm) is a well-recognised cause and survives in the intestine of cats and dogs, where it liberates ova which are then excreted in the animal's faeces. The ova form into infected larvae which can penetrate intact human skin. The feet and hands are therefore particularly prone to infection.

PAPER THREE

FURTHER READING
Chanda, J.J., Callen, J.P., and Stawiski, M.A. (1979), Malignant melanoma and its therapy: a review, *Cutis*, **23**, 759.

Clark, R.A. and Kimball, H.R. (1971), Defective granulocyte chemotaxis in Chediak–Higashi syndrome, *Journal of Clinical Investigation*, **50**, 2645.

Davis, N. (1976), Cutaneous melanoma: Queensland project, *Current Problems in Surgery*, **13**, 1.

Debois, J., Vanderpitte, J., and Degreef, H. (1978), *Yersinia enterocolitica* as a cause of erythema nodosum, *Dermatologica*, **156**, 65.

Dent, C.E. and Garretts, M. (1960), Skin changes in hypocalcaemia, *Lancet*, **i**, 142.

Eisert, J. (1965), Diabetes and diseases of the skin, *Medical Clinics of North America*, **49**, 621.

Epstein, E., Sr and Orkin, M. (1977), Scabies: clinical aspects, in *Scabies and Pediculosis*, Orkin, M. *et al.* (Eds), J B Lippincott Co., Philadelphia.

Goldin, D. and Wilkinson, D.S. (1974), Pyoderma gangrenosum with chronic myeloid leukaemia, *Proceedings of the Royal Society of Medicine*, **67**, 1239.

Greenstein, A.J., Janowitz, H.D., and Sachar, D.B. (1976), The extraintestinal complications of Crohn's disease and ulcerative colitis: a study of 700 patients, *Medicine*, **55**, 401.

Ho, V.C. and Sober, A.J. (1990), Therapy for cutaneous melanoma. An update, *Journal of the American Academy of Dermatology*, **22**, 159.

Jacobson, R.R. and Trautman, J.R. (1976), The diagnosis and treatment of leprosy, *Southern Medical Journal*, **69**, 979.

Joliffe, D.S. (1977), Leprosy reactional states and their treatment, *British Journal of Dermatology*, **97**, 345.

Katz, R., Ziegler, J., and Blank, H.E. (1965), The natural course of creeping eruption and treatment with thiabendazole, *Archives of Dermatology*, **91**, 420.

Lerner, A.B. and Nordlund, J.J. (1978), Vitiligo, *Journal of the American Medical Association*, **239**, 1183.

Magnus, K. (1977), Prognosis in malignant melanoma, *Cancer*, **40**, 389.

Mihm, M.C., Fitzpatrick, T.B., Lane-Brown, M.M., *et al.* (1973), Early detection of primary cutaneous melanoma – a color atlas, *New England Journal of Medicine*, **289**, 989.

Mitra, M.L. (1970), Vitamin-C deficiency in the elderly and its manifestations, *Journal of the American Geriatrics Society*, **18**, 67.

Perry, H.O. and Winkelmann, R.K. (1972), Bullous pyoderma gangrenosum and leukaemia, *Archives of Dermatology*, **106**, 901.

Sabin, H.K. (1966), Rothmund–Thomson syndrome: an oculocutaneous disorder, *American Journal of Diseases of Children*, **111**, 182.

Stolman, L.P., Rosenthal, D., Yaworsky, R., *et al.* (1975), Pyoderma gangrenosum and rheumatoid arthritis, *Archives of Dermatology*, **111**, 1020.

Taylor, A.M.R., Harnden, D.G., Arlett, C.F., *et al.* (1975), Ataxia telangiectasia: a human mutation with abnormal radiation sensitivity, *Nature*, **258**, 427.

Vesey, C.M. and Wilkinson, D.S. (1959), Erythema nodosum: a study of 70 cases, *British Journal of Dermatology*, **71**, 135.

PAPER FOUR

4.1. A, C, D, F, G, and H.

Comment: The vascular signs in pregnancy are a result of sustained high levels of oestrogen.

Spider naevi first appear between the second and fifth months of pregnancy and usually, but not always, clear within 3 months postpartum.

Palmar erythema is very common in pregnancy and also fades after delivery.

There is an increased incidence of Candida vulvovaginitis, as there is in the pseudo-pregnant state induced by oral contraceptives.

Herpes gestationis is a bullous eruption which may appear in a first pregnancy and, once it has occurred, inevitably develops in subsequent pregnancies. It occurs commonly in the second trimester and carries no serious risk to the mother or the fetus, though treatment may involve the use of systemic steroids, which carries with it an increased postnatal infant mortality rate.

Pruritus, usually over the abdomen, is most troublesome in the last trimester. Generalised pruritus may also occur and, if present in the last three months of pregnancy, may be due to an underlying cholestasis.

4.2. A, B, C, D, E, and G.

Comment: Tabes dorsalis is typically associated with posterior column degeneration, with ataxia, areflexia, bladder disturbances, impotence, and lancinating (lightning) pains.

Gastric or abdominal crises frequently begin with vomiting and acute abdominal pain.

Syphilitic optic atrophy is most frequently associated with tabes dorsalis and an examination of peripheral visual fields is mandatory in every suspected neurosyphilitic.

Trophic joint changes – Charcot joints – result from the loss of impairment of pain sensation. The knee joint is the most frequently involved and severe degeneration is common. Similar joint changes may be found in syringomyelia, diabetes, or spinal cord injury. The loss of deep pain also predisposes such patients to trophic ulcers on the soles (mal perforans).

The Argyll Robertson pupil is small, irregular, and does not react to light, but reacts normally to accommodation.

4.3. A, B, C, D, E, and F.

Comment: It was shown some years ago that the majority of patients with dermatitis herpetiformis have a symptomless jejunal abnormality akin to coeliac disease. The incidence varies, but at least 70% of patients show villous atrophy of the jejunum.

The jejunal mucosa shows distinctive changes, in both children and adults, with tropical sprue, Whipple's disease, amyloidosis, and eosinophilic gastro-enteritis.

Certain parasites – *Giardia lamblia* and *Coccidiodes immitis* – have also been found on jejunal biopsy.

Total villous atrophy, although characteristic, is not specific of coeliac disease. It may occur occasionally in Whipple's disease, though the diagnosis here is made by the demonstration of macrophages laden with periodic acid-Schiff staining material in the lamina propria of the intestinal wall.

In amyloidosis, deposits of amyloid may be found in the submucosa of the jejunum, especially in the arteriolar walls.

4.4. A, B, D, and F.

Comment: White nails have been associated with cirrhosis of the liver, though its incidence in practice would appear to be low. The colour change is considered to be in the nail bed and not in the nail plate.

Paired narrow white bands have been described in hypo-albuminaemia. The bands are parallel with the lunula (half-moon) and are separated from one another by areas of normal pink nail. Normality is restored when the serum albumin level is rectified.

The most characteristic nail change in Darier's disease is a white streak extending longitudinally through the nail and which may cross the lunula. Occasionally, the nails may be affected without disease elsewhere.

Yellow, and not white, nails have been associated with lymphoedema.

In chronic arsenical poisoning leuconychia occurs and are described as Mees' stripes. In *Pseudomonas pyocyanea* infection the nail plate becomes bluish-black or green in colour.

4.5. C, D, E, and F.

Comment: Rickettsia prowazekii causes epidemic typhus. *Rickettsia rickettsii* is the organism responsible for causing Rocky Mountain spotted fever (RMSF).

RMSF is transmitted by ticks such as *Dermacentor andersoni* (wood tick) and *Dermacentor variabilis* (dog tick).

The disease is ushered in with high fever, malaise, and myalgia. The rash appears 3–4 days after onset of the fever and typically consists of macules, initially on the wrists, forearms, and ankles, which become widespread within 24 hours. After 2–4 days the eruption becomes purpuric.

Major complications include myocarditis, disseminated intravascular coagulation, and central nervous system involvement.

Direct immunofluorescence of a skin biopsy, to demonstrate the presence of fluorescent organisms in the walls of the blood vessels, is the most efficient way of confirming the diagnosis.

4.6. B, C, D, and F.

Comment: The rash associated with Still's disease is seen in some 25% of patients and occurs more commonly in boys.

The lesions are non-pruritic bright pink macules or papules. They occur most commonly on the trunk and limbs, last only a few hours, and typically appear with an increase in the ambient temperature or in that of the patient.

It is more common in patients with splenomegaly, lymphadenopathy, and a raised erythrocyte sedimentation rate.

It may occur intermittently for many years and has no prognostic value.

4.7. A, B, C, D, E, and F.

Comment: Maternal infection in the first 8 weeks of pregnancy is usually responsible for the anatomical malformations that occur in the rubella syndrome. The average risk of fetal damage has been estimated as 30% for maternal infection in the first 16 weeks, 50–60% for infection acquired in the first month of gestation, and 4–5% if acquired in the fourth month.

Permanent defects include cataracts, deafness, congenital heart disease (most frequently patent ductus arteriosus), microcephaly, and mental retardation.

The infant with generalised disease may show hepatosplenomegaly, growth retardation, and purpura due to thrombocytopenia, which usually clears after a few weeks.

4.8. A, C, D, E, and G.

Comment: Refsum's syndrome, inherited as an autosomal recessive trait, consists of ichthyosis with cerebellar ataxia, deafness, and hypertrophic neuritis. The occurrence of phytanic acid in the serum, red blood cells, liver, heart, kidneys, and skeletal muscles is pathognomonic. Treatment consists of avoiding chlorophyll-containing foods.

Homocystinuria causes a malar flush, fine sparse hair, epilepsy, and mental retardation. Death from thrombo-embolic phenomena is frequent.

Acrodynia is an allergic reaction to mercury and commonly occurs in infants and children. Previously a result of mercury teething powders, now discontinued, it may still be induced by mercury-containing lotions and ointments. Restlessness and irritability are early symptoms and it is associated later with generalised erythema, with desquamation particularly of the hands and feet. When recovery occurs it is usually complete.

The metabolic defect in the Lesch–Nyhan syndrome is a lack of the enzyme hypoxanthine-guanine phosphoribosyl transferase. Spastic tetraplegia and athetosis are obvious in early childhood. The child grossly mutilates the face and hands, and typically there is partial destruction of the lower lip from self-biting.

4.9. A, B, C, D, E, and F.

Comment: Sjögren's syndrome is an auto-immune disease typified by a marked infiltration of lymphocytes and plasma cells into the lacrimal and salivary glands. This presents as dryness and atrophy of the conjunctiva and cornea – keratoconjunctivitis sicca – and a dry mouth.

It is frequently associated with rheumatoid arthritis and rheumatoid factor is present in 75–90% of cases. The disease is predominantly that of women, usually middle-aged or older.

Schirmer's test demonstrates a decreased tear secretion, which is common.

Other mucous membranes, including the nasal, gastric, vaginal, and rectal mucosae, may also show atrophy. Severe cases may therefore present with anogenital pruritus. Dryness of the skin occurs in many and may be made more conspicuous by a reduction in sweat production, because of the decrease in the number of sweat glands.

Other manifestations of Sjögren's syndrome include lymphadenopathy and hepatosplenomegaly. The pancreas may also be involved.

Antinuclear antibodies are found in up to 80% of cases. It has also been shown that some patients develop antibodies to the recently described nuclear antigens SS-A and SS-B. Of the two, SS-B has been more closely associated with the syndrome.

4.10. A, C, D, E, and G.

Comment: Idiopathic haemochromatosis is characterised by a slate-grey pigmentation of the skin, which precedes all other signs, often by many years. The pigmentation is especially prominent in the flexures and on light-exposed areas. It may also occur on the buccal mucosa, as in Addison's disease.

Primary haemochromatosis is ten times more common in males than in females.

Approximately 80% of patients develop diabetes mellitus, which is usually insulin-dependent.

The liver is enlarged, firm, and tender and there is splenomegaly in some 50% of patients. Loss of axillary and pubic hair is related to the hepatic cirrhosis and there is loss of libido with testicular atrophy.

Refractory cardiac failure and arrhythmias occur in a proportion of affected patients.

4.11. A, C, D, E, and G.

Comment: Erythema induratum, or Bazin's disease, presents as persistent or recurrent nodules, usually on the calves of women. They respond to anti-tuberculous therapy, which needs to be prolonged.

In Behçet's disease crops of small dermal nodules, resembling erythema nodosum, may appear at intervals, commonly on the legs. Characteristically, during active disease a sterile pustule develops over a site of skin puncture as may be induced for venesection purposes.

Three types of pretibial myxoedema are recognised. The first is a sharply circumscribed variety in which nodular lesions appear on the shins and toes. The second is a diffuse variety with non-pitting oedema of the shins and feet and the third is the elephantiasic variety, in which there is both oedema and nodule formation.

4.12. B, C, D, and F.

Comment: Mucous membrane lesions are exceedingly common and seen most often on the buccal mucosa and the tongue, but may also occur on the genitalia, and, rarely, even on the tympanic membrane.

The typical lesion of lichen planus is a flat, shiny, violaceous papule, on the surface of which there may often be white dots or lines known as Wickham's striae.

Annular lesions are especially common on the glans penis. The skin lesions subside within 9 months in approximately 50% of patients and within 18 months in 85%.

Alopecia in lichen planus is of the scarring variety. The inflammatory infiltrate destroys the hair follicle and patches of alopecia may continue to appear after the skin lesions have faded. The nails are involved in 10% of cases; the commonest change is a slight thinning of the nail plate, which gives rise to linear depressions on its surface.

4.13. A, C, D, F, and G.

Comment: The side-effects of oral corticosteroid therapy are akin to an iatrogenic Cushing's syndrome. Patients develop a moon face, acne, oedema, an increase in weight, striae, bruising, and mental changes.

Osteoporosis results from calcium and phosphorus depletion and fractures of ribs and vertebrae are not uncommon.

Peptic ulceration may occur and diabetes mellitus may be induced. Signs of infection can be masked and bacteria may proliferate.

Pulmonary tuberculosis may be activated and prove fatal if undiagnosed and therefore left untreated.

Corticosteroids cause sodium retention and potassium loss. An increased blood viscosity may result in venous thrombosis.

There is delayed healing of wounds due to reduced fibroblastic activity.

4.14. A, B, E, F, and G.

Comment: In hypopituitarism intolerance to cold, as in primary hypothyroidism, may be extreme.

There is loss or dimunition of axillary and pubic hair. The menses do not return or become scanty due to gonadal failure, and when hypopituitarism is due to post-partum necrosis of the pituitary, the first symptom is failure to lactate.

The skin is smooth and pale and there is a fine wrinkling around the eyes.

The breasts may appear well-preserved, but genital atrophy is the rule. Physical examination usually reveals a good nutritional state, unlike in anorexia nervosa, in which irregular menstruation is commonly associated with much loss of muscle bulk.

Pre-existing diabetes mellitus is, on rare occasions, improved abruptly, with lowering of the insulin requirement, after pituitary destruction – the Houssay phenomenon.

4.15. A, B, D, and G.

Comment: In measles the prodrome usually begins approximately 11 days after infection. The rash usually follows in 3–5 days, beginning with faint pink macules at the front hairline, in the scalp, and behind the ears. It then becomes morbilliform, extends sequentially over the face, neck, trunk, and extremities. Fading of the rash occurs in the same progression as the onset, starting on the face.

In infectious mononucleosis the rash begins in the first week of the illness proper. Typically morbilliform and most prominent over the trunk and proximal arms, it clears in a few days. Bilateral supra-orbital oedema is more common than rash and may be the presenting sign in children. In the second week 25% of patients exhibit petechiae at the junction of the hard and soft palates. A common, almost diagnostic, feature is a generalised erythematous eruption that occurs in 90% of patients within a week of receiving ampicillin.

Kaposi's varicelliform eruption is commonly caused by the herpes simplex virus, superimposed on atopic dermatitis, though any clinically diseased skin may be infected. The eruption is typified by umbilicated vesicles.

Toxic shock syndrome is an acute illness due to exotoxin-producing staphylococci. It is characterised by fever, a toxic erythema with marked desquamation of the distal extremities, hypotension (systolic blood pressure less than 90 mmHg), and multisystem involvement. Most patients are menstruating females who use tampons.

Lyme disease is a spirochetal infection caused by the treponeme *Borrelia burgdorferi*, tansmitted by the bite of the hard-bodied tick *Ixodes ricinus* in Europe and by other species elsewhere. It is typified by erythema chronicum migrans, which occurs approximately 7 days (range 3–32 days) after a tick bite. Fatigue and lethargy are often constant, whereas other symptoms and signs may be intermittent and change over time. Approximately 7% of untreated patients develop frank neurological deficits 4 weeks after a tick bite; these, if left untreated, may persist for months, but usually resolve completely. At about 5 weeks cardiac abnormalities may occur in approximately 8% of patients. The most common abnormality is AV block, to different degrees. In Lyme disease antibiotic therapy should be commenced early to stem early symptoms and signs, and to prevent recurrences and late complications. In adults oral tetracycline hydrochloride, 1 g per day for 3 weeks, is the most effective drug. In children under 8 years of age, the suggested treatment is phenoxymethylpenicillin, 1–2 g per day, or erythromycin stearate if the child is allergic to penicillin.

Hand, foot, and mouth disease is usually caused by the Coxsackie virus A16. Primarily, it affects children less than 10 years old and presents with painful vesicles and erosions in the mouth, with vesicles also over the hands and feet (hence its name). The eruption usually clears within a week.

4.16. A, B, C, and E.

Comment: Scarlet fever results from strains of *Streptococcus pyogenes*, which produce an erythrotoxin. Infection is commonest in the first decade of life and the upper respiratory tract is the usual portal of entry. By the second or third day of illness swollen red papillae are obvious on the tongue, giving it the well-described 'strawberry tongue' appearance.

The rash, a punctate erythema, appears first on the trunk on the second day. It becomes generalised within a few days and is associated with a facial flush and perioral pallor.

In severe forms of scarlet fever the eruption may be purpuric and may be associated with myocarditis. Blanching of the rash around the point of injection of antitoxin forms the basis of the Schultz–Charlton test.

A positive Dick test indicates that the subject is susceptible to scarlet fever.

4.17. A, C, F, and G.

Comment: One attack of mumps appears to confer life-long immunity. Prevention is achieved by a live attenuated mumps vaccine, which is given subcutaneously and is especially recommended for prepubertal boys who have not suffered from mumps. It should not be given to those with an allergy to egg protein or to neomycin.

Immunity after rubella infection is lasting. Haemagglutination-inhibiting (HI) antibodies against the virus have been demonstrated 30 years after the initial infection. Authenticated second attacks are rare and should be confirmed by the appropriate serologic tests. An attenuated live-virus vaccine provides immunity though, as with other live virus vaccines, serum antibody titres are lower than those that follow natural infection.

An unmodified attack of measles is usually followed by life-long immunity. Highly effective vaccines are available, though reinfection has been reported in a small number of vaccinated subjects during epidemics, presumably because of the fall in antibody titre which occurs after a few years in the absence of exposure to wild-type virus.

4.18. A, B, C, D, F, and H.

Comment: The most common cause of hypopituitarism in the adult is a pituitary tumour, particularly chromophobe adenoma. The most common cause of severe adult hypopituitarism is post-partum necrosis of the gland or Sheehan's disease.

Lesions other than tumours include granulomas, which may be non-specific or due to syphilis or tuberculosis. Ischaemic necrosis of the pituitary has also occurred after acute infection, meningitis, basal skull fracture, and septic cavernous sinus thrombosis.

In some patients the primary lesion may lie in the hypothalamus as with sarcoidosis or metastatic cancer.

Hand–Schüller–Christian disease belongs to the group of histiocytic proliferative disorders. It occurs usually between 2–6 years of age and the classical triad consists of defects in the cranial bones, exophthalmus, and diabetes insipidus due to involvement of either the pituitary stalk or the hypothalamus. Skin lesions are present in 30% of cases and may closely resemble seborrhoeic dermatitis with petechiae.

4.19. A, C, E, and F.

Comment: Secondary syphilis may present as an iritis or with constitutional symptoms, such as fever and malaise, but the diagnosis is usually suggested by the skin and mucous membrane lesions. The eruption is bilateral and symmetrical and may be macular, papular, papulosquamous, or pustular. The lesions are seldom pruritic and are usually non-vesicular.

'Moth-eaten' occipital alopecia is characteristic and may be associated with loss of eyelashes and the lateral third of the eyebrows.

Mucous patches may occur over the lips, tongue, throat, and cervix.

Treponema pallidum may be obtained from a mucous membrane or secondary cutaneous lesion, though the spirochaete is best seen in a moist lesion.

Differential diagnosis of a secondary syphilitic eruption includes pityriasis rosea, but this usually spares the head, neck, and mucous membranes, and is associated with a 'herald' patch, which precedes the eruption of pityriasis rosea by one or more weeks.

4.20. A, C, D, and E.

Comment: In the Sturge–Weber syndrome the cutaneous lesions are usually present at birth. The facial naevus is of the 'port-wine' variety and characteristically involves the trigeminal area, but may extend to the neck and trunk, and the oral mucous membrane may be involved.

Epilepsy occurs in the majority of patients and complete hemiplegia of sudden or gradual onset also develops in many.

Mental retardation has been noted in more than 60% of patients.

X-ray of the skull may show calcification in the meningeal angioma, but intracranial calcification is not always seen, especially in the early stages.

The eye is involved in many patients and may present as glaucoma or retinal detachment.

PAPER FOUR

FURTHER READING

Axelrod, L. (1976), Glucocorticoid therapy, *Medicine*, 55, 39.

Baum, G.L. and Schwarz, J. (1974), Diagnosis and treatment of systemic mycoses, *Medical Clinics of North America*, 58, 662.

Bloch, K.J., Buchanan, W.W., Wohl, M., *et al.* (1965), Sjögren's syndrome. A clinical, pathological and serological study of sixty-two cases, *Medicine*, 44, 187.

Cooper, L.Z., Green, R.H., Krugman, S., *et al.* (1965), Neonatal thrombocytopenic purpura and other manifestations of rubella contracted *in utero*, *American Journal of Diseases of Children*, 110, 416.

Feiwel, M. and Munro, D.D. (1965), Diagnosis and treatment of erythema induratum, *British Medical Journal*, 5442, 1109.

Felman, Y.M. and Nikitas, J.A. (1982), Secondary syphilis, *Cutis*, 29, 322.

Forström, L. and Hannuksela, M. (1970), Antituberculous treatment of erythema induratum Bazin, *Acta Dermatovenereologica*, 50, 143.

Helmick, L.G., Bernard, K.W., and D'Angelo, L.J. (1984), Rocky Mountain spotted fever: clinical, laboratory and epidemiological features of 262 cases, *Journal of Infectious Diseases*, 150, 480.

Isdale, I.C. and Bywaters, E.G.L. (1956), The rash of rheumatoid arthritis and Still's disease, *Quarterly Journal of Medicine*, 25, 377.

King, A. and Nicol, C. (1975), *Venereal Diseases*, 3rd edn, Bailliére-Tindall, London.

Kolodny, R.E. (1969), Herpes gestationis, *American Journal of Obstetrics and Gynecology*, 104, 39.

Lamkin, B.C. (1981), Dermatitis herpetiformis. Its relationship to gastrointestinal disease, *Cutis*, 28, 302.

Lesch, M. and Nyhan, W.L. (1964), A familial disorder of uric acid metabolism and central nervous system function, *American Journal of Medicine*, 36, 561.

Long, J.C., Mihm, M.C., and Qazi, R. (1976), Malignant lymphoma of the skin, *Cancer*, 38, 1282.

Marks, J., Shuster, S., and Watson, A.J. (1966), Small bowel changes in dermatitis herpetiformis, *Lancet*, ii, 1280.

Paterman, A.F., Hatles, A.B., Dockerty, M.B., *et al.* (1958), Encephalotrigeminal angiomatosis (Sturge–Weber disease), *Journal of the American Medical Association,* 167, 2169.

Sarkany, I. and Gaylarde, P.M. (1972), The pathogenesis of lichen planus, *British Journal of Dermatology*, 87, 81.

Saurat, J.H., Didier-Jean, L., Gluckman, E., *et al.*, (1975), Graft *versus* host reaction and lichen planus-like eruption in man, *British Journal of Dermatology*, 92, 591.

Sheehan, H.L. and Summers, V.K. (1949), The syndrome of hypopituitarism, *Quarterly Journal of Medicine*, 42, 319.

Storrs, F.J. (1979), Use and abuse of systemic corticosteroid therapy, *Journal of the American Academy of Dermatology*, 1, 95.

Talal, N. (1980), Advances in the diagnosis and concept of Sjögren's syndrome (autoimmune exocrinopathy), *Bulletin on the Rheumatic Diseases*, 30, 1046.

Wade, T.R., Wade, S.L., and Jones, H.E. (1978), Skin changes and diseases associated with pregnancy, *Obstetrics and Gynecology*, 52, 233.

PAPER FIVE

5.1. A, B, C, E, and F.

Comment: Diffuse hyperpigmentation is recognised as one of the many signs of neoplasia. In the ectopic ACTH syndrome associated with an oat-cell carcinoma of the bronchus, pigmentation is usual.

Paget's disease of the nipple is associated with an intraductal carcinoma of the breast.

Acanthosis nigricans can be a marker of underlying malignancy, particularly when it develops in adult life.

Childhood dermatomyositis is not normally associated with neoplasia, but the adult onset variety (40–60 years) is frequently found with malignancy (15–20% of patients).

Herpes zoster occurs more commonly and is more likely to be disseminated in patients with an underlying reticulosis.

5.2. A, B, C, D, E, and F.

Comment: Essential factors in the production of a trophic ulcer are loss of pain sensation and trauma. In leprosy, tabes dorsalis, spinal vascular disease, and syringomyelia there is sensory loss.

In diabetes mellitus, both peripheral neuropathy and vascular insufficiency contribute to the development of a trophic ulcer. In one series diabetes mellitus was the most frequent cause of neurotrophic ulcers of the foot.

The presence of pain does not rule out the diagnosis of a neurotrophic ulcer, as referred pain can be present in an anaesthetic ulcer.

5.3. A, B, C, E, and F.

Comment: Seborrhoeic eczema is a misnomer as there is little evidence for dysfunction or a disorder of the sebaceous glands. It usually first appears at 3–4 weeks of age and, in most instances, clears when the infant is 3–4 months old.

Miliaria (prickly heat) is often found in the napkin area because of the hot, humid conditions frequently exacerbated by a plastic-covered napkin.

Juvenile pemphigoid presents with bullae, which may be restricted to the genitalia, lower abdomen, buttocks, and face.

Acrodermatitis enteropathica due to zinc deficiency can present as an acute eczema in the napkin area, around the mouth, and over the extremities.

Letterer–Siwe disease, the malignant form of histiocytosis X, starts with an intertrigo which can mimic seborrhoeic eczema.

5.4. A, C, D, E, and F.

Comment: In tinea versicolor the pigment formed is produced by the fungus, rather than by the skin.

A diffuse grey–brown pigmentation occurs in haemochromatosis.The role of iron in stimulating melanin deposition in the disease is not clear.

The pigmentation of pregnancy is probably a result of the joint action of oestrogen and progesterone on the melanocyte.

In scleroderma pigmentation develops in almost 50% of patients. It usually occurs on the face, but occasionally it may be diffuse and suggest Addison's disease.

5.5. A, B, D, E, and F.

Comment: Candida albicans is a frequent inhabitant of the gastrointestinal tract in otherwise healthy individuals.

In hypoparathyroidism, hypothyroidism, and Cushing's syndrome increased susceptibility to candidiasis is thought to be related to depressed immune, especially T cell, function.

C. albicans is commonly isolated from the skin in a napkin eruption. The organism may be the cause of the rash, though it is frequently a secondary invader.

In fungal endocarditis, most frequently caused by Candida or Histoplasma, a characteristic is embolic occlusion of large arteries. It is suggested that this occurs because of the bulky vegetations induced by these organisms.

5.6. A, B, and C.

Comment: Cutis marmorata is a physiological reaction to cold, commonly seen on the lower limbs. It presents as a reticular vascular pattern, which clears on rewarming the skin.

Chilblains or perniosis arise as a reaction to cold, which causes constriction of arterioles and venules.

Erythema ab igne results from prolonged exposure to heat, as from a fire (igne).

5.7. A, B, C, D, and E.

Comment: Cutaneous manifestations include fair hair and skin (due to impaired melanin synthesis), eczema, which may be of the atopic variety, and dermographism. The incidence of pyogenic infection is also increased.

The enzyme phenylalanine hydroxylase, which converts phenylalanine into tyrosine, is usually absent.

A low phenylalanine diet is essential in therapy, though in some instances may safely be stopped after the first 8 years of life.

Phenylketonuria (PKU) accounts for 0.04–1% of mental defectives in institutions. The electroencephalogram is abnormal in 80% of patients with PKU.

5.8. B, C, D, E, and F.

Comment: Chloasma or melasma is seen in 10–15% of women who receive synthetic progesterones and oestrogens for birth control.

In some women diffuse hair shedding – telogen effluvium – occurs 3 or 4 weeks after the contraceptive has been discontinued.

Herpes gestationis is a bullous disease of pregnancy. It usually occurs in the second or third trimester of pregnancy or in the puerperium, and recurs in successive pregnancies. It may also recur with the use of an oral contraceptive.

5.9. B, C, E, and F.

Comment: Herpes zoster occurs most frequently on the thoracic dermatomes, both in children and adults.

Anthrax, or the malignant pustule, is caused by *Bacillus anthracis*. It occurs commonly on exposed skin, in particular of the hands and face.

Lichen sclerosus is seen most frequently on the genitalia.

Erysipeloid is caused by the organism *Erysipelothrix insidiosa*, and is a hazard for those who handle animal carcasses – cooks, butchers, and veterinary surgeons, though housewives may be infected if the skin is pierced by an infected fish or chicken bone.

5.10. A, B, and C.

Comment: Diabetes mellitus, psoriasis, and acne vulgaris are considered to have a polygenic mode of inheritance.

Twin studies provide evidence that psoriasis is hereditary, but the mode of inheritance remains speculative, since it is difficult to distinguish between multifactorial inheritance and two alleles at a single locus, on the basis of empirical data alone.

Acne shows a distinct familial bias and is commoner in certain races. In one survey, almost five out of ten boys with acne had one or both parents who had also suffered from acne, whereas less than one in ten boys without acne had a parent with a history of acne.

5.11. A, C, and E.

Comment: Sporotrichosis is a chronic lymphatic or subcutaneous fungal infection caused by *Sporothrix schenkii*. The fungus is usually introduced into the skin by minor injury and is characterised by lymphatic involvement, which results in a chain of nodules.

Linear morphoea occurs commonly in children and may involve an entire limb. Atrophy of muscle and subcutaneous tissue can cause contracture and shortening of the affected limb.

5.12. A, B, C, D, E, and F.

Comment: HIV-1 was first isolated in 1983 and HIV-2, related to but distinct from HIV-1, was first identified in 1985. It is a member of the lentivirus group of the retroviridae. These viruses are characterised by a life-long persistence in their host and a long period of latency before they induce clinical signs.

The acute infection may be asymptomatic or cause an illness like that of glandular fever.

The normal T-helper cell count of approximately 800/mm^3 falls as the symptomatic phase of HIV infection begins.

The main routes of infection are sexual, administration of blood, injection with blood-contaminated equipment, and from mother to fetus. It is estimated that 20–50% of infants born to HIV-infected mothers will be infected.

5.13. A, B, C, D, E, F, and G.

Comment: The multiplicity of causes of gynaecomastia reflects the complex hormonal mechanisms responsible for breast enlargement. Some breast enlargement occurs at puberty in about 60% of boys.

Patients with testicular teratoma often have a high serum concentration of human chorionic gonadotrophin (HCG), which stimulates oestrogen production. Other non-endocrine tumours that produce HCG are hepatoma and large-cell bronchial carcinoma (10% of cases).

When drug-related, withdrawal of the offending drug reduces the discomfort associated with gynaecomastia. In the majority of symptomatic patients an anti-oestrogen, such as tamoxifen, or a gonadotrophin inhibitor, such as danazol, is useful.

5.14. A, B, C, D, and E.

Comment: Tinea versicolor is a mild chronic fungal infection of the skin. It is caused by the conversion of a normal saprophyte of skin, *Pityrosporon orbiculare,* into the pathogenic form, *Malassezia furfur.*

The term versicolor implies a change from one colour to another; in dark skin tinea versicolor may appear as whitish patches and be mistaken for vitiligo, whilst in fair skin it can present as brown macules. When viewed under a Wood's lamp (long-wave ultraviolet light) it fluoresces a golden yellow.

5.15. A, B, C, D, E, and F.

Comment: In clubbing increased fibrous tissue separates the nail from the phalanx. In cyanotic congenital heart disease, clubbing is seldom noticeable before the second year of life, whereas in malignant pulmonary disease the onset may be rapid and painful. The pathogenesis of clubbing of the fingers remains uncertain, but a low arterial oxygen tension and increased blood flow cannot account for all the cases encountered.

In ulcerative colitis clubbing is rare in the absence of co-existing small bowel involvement.

5.16. B, C, D, E, F, and G.

Comment: Peyronie's disease is a chronic fibrous induration of the intercavernous septa of the penis. Ulceration is not a feature, but there is a well-described association with Dupuytren's contracture.

In Reiter's disease penile lesions occur in approximately 25% of patients. In the uncircumcised male moist erosions develop and coalesce to form the so called 'circinate balanitis'.

Pemphigus vulgaris, a disorder characterised by the formation of intra-epithelial bullae, commonly involves the genitalia. The bullae rupture easily and leave ulcerated inflamed areas.

5.17. A, B, C, and D.

Comment: The frequency of metastases to the skin varies from 1–4.5%. The scalp is a common site for metastases from the breast, lung, and genito-urinary cancers.

Discoid lupus erythematosus characteristically produces inflammatory plaques on the face, arms, and trunk. Lesions of the scalp invariably result in scarring alopecia.

Lichen planus of the scalp is seen more frequently in women, especially between the ages of 30–60 years.

Alopecia areata and cyclophosphamide-induced hair loss are causes of non-scarring alopecia.

5.18. A, B, C, E, and F.

Comment: Pigmentation is present in most patients and commonly seen as well-defined brown patches, often 2–5 cm in length.

Axillary freckling is considered to be pathognomonic and is found in 20% of patients.

Neurological manifestations are found in some 40% of patients and the commonest solitary intracranial tumour is an optic nerve glioma. Astrocytomas and schwannomas also occur.

Sarcomatous change within a neurofibroma arises in 5–15% of cases.

Neurofibromatosis is inherited as an autosomal dominant trait with an incidence estimated at one in 2500–3000 births.

Endocrine abnormalities which may be associated include precocious puberty, hyperparathyroidism, Addison's disease, and acromegaly.

5.19. A, B, C, D, E, F, and G.

Comment: Trichinosis is caused by a round worm, *Trichinella spiralis*. Generalised pruritus can occur at the stage of muscle invasion by the parasite.

Pruritus is seen more commonly with the lymphatic rather than the granulocytic variety of leukaemia.

The pruritus of chronic renal failure has been related to the levels of blood urea and skin surface urea, and to the dryness of the skin. In many, parathyroidectomy relieves the pruritus suggesting that secondary hyperparathyroidism may also be relevant.

Pruritus occurs in some 30% of patients with Hodgkin's disease.

In biliary cirrhosis generalised pruritus can precede all other signs and may occur 1–2 years before the onset of jaundice.

A low serum iron level has been correlated with pruritus.

5.20. A, B, C, D, E, and F.

Comment: In lichen planus mucous membrane lesions are very common and occur in 30–70% of cases. The buccal mucosa and tongue are most often involved.

In the Peutz–Jeghers syndrome pigmented macules develop on the oral mucosa in association with perioral pigmentation.

In chronic discoid lupus erythematosus, lesions within the mouth are commonly seen on the palate and buccal mucosa.

In pemphigoid, bullae occur in the mouth in 20% of patients and usually late in the course of the disease.

PAPER FIVE

FURTHER READING

Beare, J.M. (1976), Generalised pruritus: a study of 43 cases, *Clinical and Experimental Dermatology*, 1, 343.

Bessman, S.P. (1964), Some biochemical lessons to be learned from phenylketonuria, *Journal of Paediatrics*, 64, 828.

Brandrup, F., Hange, M., Hennington, K., and Eriksen, B. (1978), Psoriasis in an unselected series of twins, *Archives of Dermatology*, 114, 874.

Braunstein, G.D., Vaitukaitis, J.L., Carbone, P.P., and Ross, G.T. (1973), Ectopic production of human chorionic gonadotrophin by neoplasms, *Annals of Internal Medicine*, 78, 39.

Buckle, R. (1977), Studies on the treatment of gynaecomastia with danazol (Danol), *Journal of International Medical Research*, 5 (Supplement 3), 114.

Cohen, R., Roth, F.J., Delgado, E., Ahearn, D.G., and Kalser, M.H. (1969), Fungal flora of the normal human small and large intestine, *New England Journal of Medicine*, 280, 638.

Edwards, J.E. (1978), Severe candidal infections: clinical perspective, immune defence mechanisms and current concepts of theory, *Annals of Internal Medicine*, 89, 91.

Ewer, R.W., Antes, E.H., and Brakel, F.J. (1963), Tape test for acquired hyperkeratosis of skin with pigmentation: with special reference to patients with cancer, *Archives of Internal Medicine*, 111, 634.

Fischer, D.S., Singer, D., and Feldman, S.M. (1964), Clubbing. A review with emphasis on hereditary acropachy, *Medicine (Baltimore)*, 43, 459.

Griffiths, W.A.D. (1973), Diffuse hair loss and oral contraceptives, *British Journal of Dermatology*, 88, 31.

Hovig, D.E., Hodgman, J.E., and Mathies, S.W. (1968), Herpesvirus hominis (simplex) infection in the newborn, *American Journal of Diseases of Children*, 115, 438.

Jefferys, D.B. (1979), Painful gynaecomastia treated with tamoxifen, *British Medical Journal*, 1, 1119.

Kelly, P.J. and Coventry, M.B. (1958), Neurotrophic ulcers of the feet, *Journal of the American Medical Association*, 168, 388.

Mitchell, D.M. (1966), Herpes gestationis and the 'pill', *British Medical Journal*, 2, 1324.

Montes, L.F., Pitillo, R.F., Hunt, D., Narkates, A.J., and Dillon, H.C. (1971), Microbial flora of infant's skin, *Archives of Dermatology*, 103, 400.

Montgomery, H. and Kierland, R.R. (1940), Metastases of carcinoma to the scalp, *Archives of Surgery*, 40, 672.

Moynahan, E.J. (1974), Acrodermatitis enteropathica: a lethal inherited skin disorder, *Lancet*, ii, 399.

Perry, H.O. and Mayne, J.G. (1965), Psoriasis and Reiter's syndrome, *Archives of Dermatology*, 92, 129.

Price, J. (1965), Two cases of heel ulceration with contralateral infarction of the sensory pathway, *Gerontologia Clinica*, 7, 115.

Robertson, A.F. and Sotos, J. (1975), Treatment of acrodermatitis enteropathica with zinc sulfate, *Pediatrics*, 55, 738.

Rothfield, H., March, C.H., Miescher, P., and Mcewen, C. (1963), Chronic discoid lupus erythematosus. A study of 65 patients and 65 controls, *New England Journal of Medicine*, **269**, 1155.

Shanbrom, E., Miller, S., and Haar, H. (1960), Herpes zoster in haematologic neoplasias: some unusual manifestations, *Annals of Internal Medicine*, **53**, 523.

Smith, C. (1971), Discriminating between different modes of inheritance in genetic disease, *Clinical Genetics*, **2**, 303.

Smith, C., Falconer, D.S., and Duncan, L.J.P. (1972), A statistical and genetical study of diabetes. II. Hereditability of liability, *Annals of Human Genetics*, **35**, 281.

Vickers, C.F.H. (1973), Iron deficiency and the skin, *British Journal of Dermatology*, Supplement 9, 10.

PAPER SIX

6.1. B, C, D, and E.

Comment: Pyoderma gangrenosum typically presents as a tender nodule that ulcerates. The common sites for the lesions are the calves, thighs, and buttocks. The ulcer crater usually has a necrotic base, an irregular bluish-purple edge (gangrenosum), and a surrounding halo of erythema. After appropriate therapy it heals with atrophy. Enlargement of the ulcer can be rapid, however, and the lesion may extend several centimetres in a few days.

Pyoderma gangrenosum was first associated with ulcerative colitis, with 80% of patients in the original classic description having ulcerative colitis.

The onset and severity of the skin lesions often parallel the activity of the bowel disease.

Pyoderma gangrenosum is frequently associated with systemic disease, but may occur without associated disease in patients who have been in good health.

6.2. B, C, and E.

Comment: Rabies does not produce skin lesions, although the patient may suffer intermittent pain, tingling, or bruising around the site of infection. Hyperaesthesia of the skin may also occur, being provoked by temperature changes or draughts.

Molluscum contagiosum is mildly contagious and auto-inoculation does occur. The lesions are dome-shaped umbilicated papules, which clear on piercing with a sharpened orange stick dipped in podophyllin.

Rocky Mountain spotted fever is a self-limiting rickettsial infection.

Orf is a viral infection of sheep and goats which is occasionally transmitted to man. A papule forms, commonly on the fingers, hands, or face, then develops into a large vesicle or haemorrhagic bulla, and heals within 4–6 weeks.

6.3. A, B, C, D, E, F, and G.

Comment: Late congenital syphilis is an ante-natally acquired infection which has persisted and developed in children over the age of 2 years. Residual features of early lesions may be present, such as rhagades around the mouth and bowing of the tibia from periostitis.

One of the characteristic stigmas is deformity of the upper incisors. They become wedge-shaped, widely spaced, and often notched (Hutchinson's teeth).

Eighth nerve deafness occurs rarely, but is usually bilateral and not influenced by anti-syphilitic treatment.

The most common affliction is interstitial keratitis, which usually becomes apparent in late childhood and eventually becomes bilateral: vision is impaired and patients exhibit photophobia.

Other late manifestations include meningovascular syphilis, paresis, and tabes, but cardiovascular complications are rare.

6.4. A and B.

Comment: Maculopapular skin lesions usually appear by the second week of the illness, but can occur as late as the end of the third week. Their incidence varies between 50–90% of patients, although generally it is seen less frequently in children.

The 'rose spots' are usually found on the abdomen and chest, and are rarely seen on the face, hands, or feet. The lesions appear in crops over a period of 1–2 weeks; individual lesions last for 3–4 days.

Salmonella typhi can be isolated from the blood in approximately 90% of patients in the first week of illness and in about 50% at the end of the third week.

Intestinal haemorrhage may occur during the second or third week of illness. Perforation, usually in the lower ileum, occurs in approximately 1% of patients. Cholecystectomy terminates the chronic enteric carrier stage in about 85% of patients.

Chloramphenicol therapy has not been shown to be effective for chronic carriers and is not recommended.

6.5. A, B, C, D, E, and F.

Comment: Seborrhoeic eczema, now considered to be the result of an overgrowth or hypersensitivity to Pityrosporum yeasts, is one of the commonest signs in HIV disease. It is seen in more than 50% of AIDS patients, and usually responds to topical imidazoles alone or combined with a topical steroid.

Itchy folliculitis usually presents as an eruption of small very pruritic papules on the head, neck, and trunk that are virtually resistant to oral antimicrobials, oral antihistamines, and topical anti-inflammatory agents, although some patients obtain relief with ultraviolet light or psoralen with long-wave ultraviolet light (PUVA) therapy.

Drug reactions are common in AIDS, particularly with sulphonamides which result in a maculopapular eruption within 1–2 weeks of treatment, as well as in urticaria, erythema multiforme, and toxic epidermal necrolysis.

Molluscum contagiosum infection, particularly of the face, is common and highly characteristic of HIV disease.

6.6. A, B, D, and E.

Comment: Lupus vulgaris is a post-primary tuberculous infection of the skin.

The typical lesion is a plaque composed of nodules which show an 'apple jelly' colour on diascopy. If untreated, the disease spreads; the older the patient at the onset of the lesions, the more rapid the spread.

The nasal or conjunctival mucosa may be involved and nasal lesions may invade or destroy the cartilage.

Bacilli are cultured infrequently and in one large series were demonstrated in only 6% of nearly 4000 patients.

Squamous cell and, less commonly, basal cell carcinomata may occur in plaques of lupus vulgaris, usually after the disease has been present for at least 10 years.

6.7. A, C, D, and F.

Comment: Raynaud's phenomenon, without any apparent reason, affects the hands more often than the feet.

A typical attack consists of sudden pallor in one or more fingers, followed by cyanosis and then erythema.

In severe cases telangiectasia of the nail folds, thinning of the nails, and sclerosis and atrophy of the fingers may result.

In Raynaud's phenomenon secondary to occlusive arterial disease asymmetrical involvement of digits occurs. A cervical rib is an uncommon though recognised cause.

Aperistalsis of the oesophagus may occur in 'uncomplicated' Raynaud's phenomenon or secondary to lupus erythematosus, systemic sclerosis, or dermatomyositis.

6.8. B, D, E, and G.

Comment: In rheumatoid arthritis a globulin called the rheumatoid factor is produced. The latex fixation tube test is the most widely used method for detecting rheumatoid factor. The sensitivity in well-established cases of adult rheumatoid arthritis is about 75%, with normal controls showing a positive test in approximately 1% of cases. The latex test may also be positive in collagen vascular diseases, such as systemic lupus erythematosus, sarcoidosis, syphilis, cirrhosis, and hepatitis.

In Sjögren's syndrome rheumatoid factor tests are positive in the majority of patients.

Felty's syndrome consists of rheumatoid arthritis, splenomegaly, and neutropenia. Rheumatoid factor is invariably positive and antinuclear factor is more commonly found than in uncomplicated rheumatoid arthritis.

6.9. B, C, D, and E.

Comment: Streptococcal tonsillitis or otitis media may precipitate guttate psoriasis in children; this has long been recognised.

Vaccination may also occasionally provoke psoriasis.

Acute guttate attacks may also follow childbirth, but pre-existing psoriasis is more commonly improved rather than worsened during pregnancy.

Hypocalcaemia has been associated with pustular psoriasis; in some cases of generalised pustular psoriasis (Zumbusch) it appears to have preceded relapses and may be causally related.

6.10. A, C, D, and F.

Comment: The characteristic skin eruption has features of both annular erythema and toxic epidermal necrolysis; it has been labelled 'necrolytic migratory erythema'. The triad of chronic superficial necrolytic dermatosis, a smooth shiny tongue, and hyperglycaemia has been termed 'a pancreatic dermatosis'. The typical skin rash, anaemia, and diabetes have together been called the 'glucagonoma syndrome'.

The eruption is chronic, with spontaneous remissions and exacerbations; it may also simulate various dermatoses, such as pemphigus vulgaris, toxic epidermal necrolysis, and acrodermatitis enteropathica.

It does not respond to antibiotic therapy.

The islet cell tumour responsible for the syndrome is composed of glucagon-secreting alpha cells, and is usually situated in the body or tail of the pancreas. In one series, in four out of 25 cases the skin cleared after resection of the pancreatic tumour. When metastases are present, a nitrosurea derivative, streptozocin (which impairs the pancreatic production of glucagon), is helpful in some patients.

6.11. A, B, D, and F.

Comment: Senile purpura occurs because of the lack of connective tissue support of the blood vessels. The vascular fragility results in purpura or small bruises after minor trauma, although it may appear spontaneously. The lesions are painless and may persist for several weeks. The only laboratory abnormality is a positive tourniquet test (Hess' test) in some patients. There is no effective treatment. Corticosteroids produce purpura for similar reasons.

Purpura has also been reported to occur in approximately 20% of patients with malnutrition. Occasional cases of non-thrombocytopenic purpura have been reported with hyperglobulinaemia. This may be idiopathic or secondary to sarcoid, lupus erythematosus, or cirrhosis. The mechanism for the development of purpura is uncertain.

6.12. A, B, C, D, F, and H.

Comment: Cushing's syndrome results from excess glucocorticoid production by the adrenal cortex. Many of the major changes in Cushing's can be related to the known actions of cortisol. Prolonged high concentrations of cortisol result in accelerated protein catabolism, and this protein wasting together with increased capillary fragility causes easy bruising.

Striae form in areas where fatty tissue accumulates.

Cortisol impairs antibody production and lymphocyte proliferation, which allows infections to spread more easily; those such as tinea versicolor may become widespread.

Adrenal carcinomas that secrete cortisol may also produce androgen. In women this may present as acne, thinning of scalp hair, or facial hirsutism.

Pigmentation of an Addisonian pattern develops in some 10% of patients; its presence suggests a pituitary tumour.

6.13. A, B, C, and F.

Comment: Secondary amyloidosis, unlike primary amyloidosis, is secondary to an underlying disease; treatment of the cause may lead to a regression of the amyloid deposits, which occur typically in the kidneys, liver, the spleen, and the adrenals.

Secondary amyloidosis may result from tuberculosis, rheumatoid arthritis, lepromatous leprosy, and osteomyelitis.

Skin diseases, such as hidradenitis suppurativa, dystrophic epidermolysis bullosa, and chronic leg ulcers, are other recognised causes.

The diagnosis has usually been made by rectal biopsy, but more recently biopsy of normal skin, which includes subcutaneous fat, has been recommended as equally suitable.

6.14. A, B, D, E, and F.

Comment: Mast cell disease in infancy may present as a solitary tumour, a widespread maculopapular eruption, a bullous eruption, or as a diffuse infiltration of the skin. All of these forms may be associated with systemic signs and symptoms.

Systemic mastocytosis also refers to the disease when it affects organs other than the skin. The liver, spleen, lymph nodes, bone marrow, and gastro-intestinal tract may be infiltrated with mast cells.

Dermographism may be illustrated on normal skin; rubbing a typical lesion may also cause it to wheal – Darier's sign.

Peptic ulcers may form, and are believed to result from the release of excessive amounts of histamine from the mast cells.

Bone lesions may be seen on X-ray as cysts, osteosclerosis, or thickening of body trabeculae.

6.15. A, C, D, and E.

Comment: Porphyria cutanea tarda (PCT) is the most frequently encountered porphyria. The disease is more common in males and usually occurs in the fifth or sixth decades in life.

Alcoholism is common in PCT, but it is not essential for its development. However, treatment in the past consisted simply of stopping alcohol consumption; this alone resulted in a remission in 50% of patients.

Increased fragility of the skin, with blister and scar formation, especially on the dorsa of the hands, are significant clinical findings.

Increased deposition of iron in the liver is frequently found and serum iron is usually elevated.

There is no increase in faecal protoporphyrin, as in porphyria variegata.

6.16. A, B, C, and F.

Comment: The syndrome of kwashiorkor presents with a pitting oedema, usually of the lower limbs, but which may be generalised in severe cases.

The changes in the skin are typically akin to those in pellagra.

The dermatitic lesions, which pigment, appear to be most numerous on areas prone to friction, especially over the perineum.

Normally curly hair becomes dry, brittle, and is easily pulled out. The hair may become reddish, or even white. Alopecia is a common occurrence.

Diarrhoea is virtually a constant finding and a low total serum protein is invariable. It is almost entirely due to a low level of albumin.

6.17. True: A, B, and C.

In the first year of maternal syphilis infection most pregnancies will terminate in fetal death if the mother is left without treatment. Later in the course of the infection the risk decreases and untreated syphilitic women may give birth to healthy children.

Adequate treatment of the mother before the 18th week of gestation prevents infection of the fetus. After the 18th week, the Langhan's cell layer of the early placenta atrophies and allows the treponeme to cross the placenta to infect the fetus.

As penicillin will cross the placenta in adequate amounts, treatment of the mother after the 18th week of pregnancy will also cure the infected fetus.

6.18. A, B, C, D, and F.

Comment: Suboccipital and post-auricular and cervical lymphadenopathy may be apparent up to a week before the rash appears, but their absence does not exclude the diagnosis and neither is their presence pathognomonic of rubella.

The rash appears first on the face, and then spreads rapidly to the trunk and limbs. On the second day the face begins to clear, by the third day the trunk has cleared, and by the fourth the eruption over the limbs has faded.

The rash may be absent in some 40% of cases.

In adults, arthritis has been reported to occur in 30% of women and 5% of men. The small or large joints may be involved.

6.19. A, D, E, and F.

Comment: Prolonged high doses of chlorpromazine and related phenothiazines cause pigmentary changes in the skin, which range from tan to slate blue or purple. Antimalarials also alter skin colour. Mepacrine produces a diffuse yellowish discolouration, while chloroquine may whiten hair and at the same time stain the skin a bluish-grey colour.

Hydantoin can produce a chloasma-like pigmentation, which fades within a few months of the drug being stopped.

Busulfan causes a diffuse brown pigmentation in 5–10% of patients.

Other antimitotic drugs, such as bleomycin and cyclophosphamide, also produce increased skin pigmentation.

6.20. A, B, D, and F.

Comment: Sexual precocity occurs some three times more frequently in girls than in boys. Precocious puberty may be caused by organic lesions of the brain that involve, either directly or indirectly, the posterior hypothalamus; these may be caused by craniopharyngioma, tuberous sclerosis, and neurofibromatosis.

Albright's syndrome includes sexual precocity, pigmentation of skin, and polyostotic fibrous dysplasia. The full syndrome occurs almost exclusively in females. It seems likely that the early puberty is not due to the premature release of pituitary gonadotrophins, but that the cause may lie in the ovary itself.

Other ovarian abnormalities, particularly granulosa cell tumours may present with sexual precocity. In boys, sexual precocity due to pinealoma is well recognised, and is probably due to ectopic chorionic gonadotrophin production by the tumour. Similar ectopic chorionic gonadotrophin production has been noted in hepatoblastoma and orchidoblastoma.

PAPER SIX

FURTHER READING

Burgoon, C.F., Graham, J.H., and McCaffere, D.L. (1968), Mast cell disease. A cutaneous variant with multisystem involvement, *Archives of Dermatology*, 98, 590.

Caplan, R.M. (1963), The natural course of urticaria pigmentosum, *Archives of Dermatology*, 87, 146.

Denko, C.W. and Zumpft, C.W. (1962), Chronic arthritis with splenomegaly and leukopenia, *Arthritis and Rheumatism*, 5, 479.

Editorial (1975), Amyloidosis and leprosy, *Lancet*, ii, 589.

Epstein, J.H. and Pinski, J.B. (1965), Porphyria cutanea tarda, *Archives of Dermatology*, 92, 362.

Fry, L. (1968), The nature of psoriasis, *British Journal of Dermatology*,80, 833.

Gilman, R.H., Terminel, M., Levine, M.M., *et al.* (1975), Relative efficacy of blood, urine, rectal swab, bone-marrow and rose-spot cultures for recovery of Salmonella typhi in typhoid fever, *Lancet*, i, 1211.

Granstein, R.D. (1981), Drug and heavy metal-induced hyperpigmentation, *Journal of the American Academy of Dermatology*, 5, 1.

Grant, D.B. (1980), Variations in the clinical and endocrine patterns of female precocious puberty, in *Pathophysiology of Puberty*, Cacciari, E. and Prader, A. (Eds), London, Academic Press, p. 175.

Levantine, A. and Almeyda, J. (1973), Drug induced changes in pigmentation, *British Journal of Dermatology*, 89, 105.

Litwack, K., Hoke, A.W., and Borchardt, K.A. (1972), Rose spots in typhoid fever, *Archives of Dermatology*, 105, 252.

Lugt, L., van der (1965), Some remarks about tuberculosis of the skin and tuberculids, *Dermatologica*, 131, 266.

Mallinson, C.N., Bloom, S.R., Warin, A.P., *et al.* (1974), A glucagonoma syndrome, *Lancet*, ii, 1.

Oppenheimer, E.H. and Hardy, J.B. (1971), Congenital syphilis in the newborn infant: clinical and pathological observations in recent cases, *John Hopkins Medical Journal*, 129, 63.

Porter, J.M., Bardana, E.J., Bauer, G.M., *et al.* (1976), The clinical significance of Raynaud's syndrome, *Surgery*, 80, 756.

Roseberg, E.W. and Yusk, J.W. (1970), Molluscum contagiosum, *Archives of Dermatology*, 101, 439.

Stein, I.F. and Leventhal, M.L. (1935), Amenorrhoea associated with bilateral polycystic ovaries, *American Journal of Obstetrics and Gynecology*, 29, 181.

Whyte, H.J. and Baugman, R.D. (1974), Acute guttate psoriasis and streptococcal infection, *Archives of Dermatology*, 89, 350.

PAPER SEVEN

7.1. A, B, D, and E.

Comment: A syndrome indistinguishable from systemic lupus erythematosus (SLE) has been reported following treatment with procainamide, hydralazine, isoniazid, and phenytoin. The development of SLE with these drugs appears to be dose-related.

SLE should only be considered to be drug-induced if it can be shown that the disease clearly followed administration of the drug, regressed on cessation of the drug, and recurred with resumption of the drug.

Laboratory findings include lupus erythematous (LE) cells, antinuclear antibodies, and antibodies to single-stranded DNA (and only very rarely those to double-stranded DNA). In drug-induced LE, renal and central nervous system involvement is rare.

7.2. A, B, C, and E.

Comment: Kaposi's sarcoma is regarded as multifocal rather than metastasising, and early histological changes can be detected in clinically unaffected skin.

In most cases its course is insidious, although occasionally it may behave aggressively, with lung involvement as the cause of death.

The usual presentation is with skin lesions, but involvement of internal organs and widespread lymphadenopathy is common; in one study visceral lesions alone were reported at post-mortem in some 30% of cases.

The skin lesions are red or purplish macules, nodules, or plaques distributed over any part of the body, but common sites are the tip of the nose and the hard palate. Lesions may also exhibit the Köebner phenomenon.

The tumours are sensitive to radiotherapy and, for many lesions, single-dose radiotherapy may be sufficient.

7.3. A, B, C, E, and F.

Comment: Palmar erythema, seen best over the thenar and hypothenar eminences, is due to local vasodilatation with increased blood flow. It occurs in pregnancy, cirrhosis, and rheumatoid arthritis.

Palmar erythema with or without spider naevi may also be acquired as an autosomal dominant trait.

Cinchona, obtained from the dried bark of several varieties of cultivated cinchona trees, contains quinine. The repeated administration of quinine in full therapeutic doses may cause cinchonism, which is characterised by tinnitus, nausea, headache, abdominal pain, disturbed vision, and often urticaria.

7.4. A, C, D, and E

Comment: It is generally agreed that griseofulvin should be taken after food, which is thought to influence the transit time of other gut contents.

Griseofulvin is fungistatic. It has no activity against bacteria or yeasts.

When warfarin and griseofulvin are given together a careful monitoring of prothrombin levels is necessary; when the antifungal is stopped the warfarin dose should also be reduced promptly.

7.5. A, B, C, E, and G.

Comment: In primary biliary cirrhosis xanthomas usually appear over the trunk, face, and extremities. Extensive plane xanthomas may develop on the hands.

Secondary xanthomatosis also occurs in hypothyroidism, the nephrotic syndrome, and some cases of diabetes.

In multiple myeloma and haemochromatosis the xanthomas are usually of the plane variety. Deposits of lipid, mainly cholesterol, are absorbed by macrophages in the dermis or subcutaneous tissue.

7.6. A, B, C, E, and F.

Comment: Raynaud's phenomemon is recognised as a paroxysmal ischaemia of the fingers and toes that is induced by cold and often relieved by heat. The affected digits blanch on exposure to cold, then turn cyanotic, and finally become a bright red colour as a result of reactive hyperaemia.

Raynaud's phenomenon may precede the development of systemic sclerosis by several years.

With long-standing Raynaud's phenomenon trophic changes appear. The skin of the fingers becomes less supple, the finger pulp mass diminishes, and areas of gangrene may appear on the finger tips. Treatment is directed at the cause, but sympathectomy and low molecular weight dextran both have their advocates for cases provoked by trauma and systemic sclerosis.

7.7. A, B, C, D, E, and F.

Comment: Measles-induced viraemia provokes a cell-mediated (T cell) response. This results in a temporary suppression of tuberculin sensitivity and an increased susceptibility to tuberculosis. For similar reasons a remission in eczema, leukaemia, or Hodgkin's disease may occur.

Meningo-encephalitis is the typical complication of the nervous system. It occurs between the fifth and tenth day of illness and nearly always before the rash has cleared. The onset may be abrupt, with convulsions, or insidious, with the child feeling lethargic or drowsy. As with other post-infectious encephalitides, such as after mumps or varicella, the pathological picture in measles-induced encephalitis is a perivascular demyelinisation of the white matter of the brain.

7.8. B, C, and E.

Comment: Co-trimoxazole is useful in the treatment of acne; it is used when the most commonly employed anti-acne drug, tetracycline, has failed to produced a satisfactory improvement.

Iodides and bromides may provoke an acute acneiform eruption and also exacerbate existing acne.

Isoniazid also causes an acneiform eruption, particularly in slow inactivators of the drug. A feature of the eruption is the presence of horny plugs in pilosebaceous follicles of the face.

ACTH produces sebaceous gland hypertrophy in prepubertal boys and in women of any age. 'Steroid acne' consists of multiple pustules with little or no associated inflammation.

7.9. A, B, C, D, E, and F.

Comment: Skin lesions develop in about 10% of patients with brucellosis. Ulcerating nodules of the legs have been reported, and direct contact with *Brucella suis* in the secretions of an infected animal may convert a simple abrasion into an indolent ulcer.

Cutaneous leishmaniasis results from the bite of a sandfly. The most common site of the lesion is the face, followed by the arms and legs. A typical 'sore' slowly forms into a nodule and eventually a shallow ulcer.

Pyoderma gangrenosum, a non-infective ulceration of the skin, is a recognised complication of ulcerative colitis and is seen especially on the calves and thighs.

In sickle-cell anaemia chronic ulcers of the legs, overlying the malleoli, may occur at puberty or later.

7.10. A, B, C, and F.

Comment: Insect bite reactions are rare in the first year of life as few children have acquired by then a specific sensitivity to insect antigens. The lesions are often grouped in clusters and the common causes world-wide are fleas and bedbugs.

Urticaria can mimic insect bites; in particular, cholinergic urticaria, in which multiple small weals occur with sweating.

Campbell de Morgan spots, or cherry angiomas, are frequently seen on the trunk in the middle-aged or elderly. Commonly, they are not grouped and their number appears to vary with the environmental temperature.

7.11. A, B, C, D, and F.

Comment: The taut skin of the face in systemic sclerosis causes both 'beaking' of the nose and radial furrowing around the mouth. The constricted skin may also interfere with lip movement and prevent adequate dental hygiene.

The patient with acrosclerosis may present with transient or fixed oedema of the hands prior to the development of sclerodermatous changes.

The fingers may shorten through progressive resorption of the terminal phalanges.

Mat-like telangiectasia are commonly found on the face and hands.

Short stature is a feature of progeria, a syndrome typified by premature atherosclerosis, in which sclerodermatous skin changes and baldness occur.

7.12. A, B, C, and D.

Comment: The Köebner, or isomorphic, phenomenon is the development of a dermatosis at the site of non-specific trauma to the skin. The trauma must involve both the epidermis and the dermal papillae, and may be in the form of an operation wound, sunburn, or vaccination. The phenomenon is seen particularly in psoriasis, eczema, and lichen planus.

Viral warts can also exhibit the Köebner response; lesions over the scalp are especially likely to spread after trauma by combing or scratching.

7.13. A, C, D, E, F, and G.

Comment: Some patients with systemic lupus erythematosus (SLE) are unduly sensitive to light in the UVB (290–320 nm) range and, following a brief exposure to the sun, can develop generalised disease.

Chronic discoid lupus erythematosus (DLE) is not a feature of SLE and, in the vast majority, is a disease restricted to the skin. When chronic DLE patients develop systemic features these are often temporary.

The most quoted cutaneous feature of SLE is the 'butterfly rash' though its incidence varies from 39% in one series (Estes and Christian, 1971) to 68% in another (Grigor *et al.*, 1978). In the latter series cutaneous vasculitis, including palmar vasculitis, occurred in 70% and purpura in 24% of cases.

Scarring alopecia may occur in SLE and leg ulcers are noted in approximately 10% of patients.

7.14. A, D, and E.

Comment: Koplik's spots are small, bluish-white specks which appear on the buccal mucosa on the second day of illness. They have been likened to grains of salt on an erythematous base. When few in number they are most frequently seen in the region of the papilla of Stenson's duct – opposite the premolar teeth. Koplik's spots are absent in 5–10% of cases.

The measles (syn. morbilli) exanthem develops on the fourth day and consists of fine discrete macules.

The rash starts at the junction of the face and scalp and spreads rapidly within 24 hours to the rest of the face, the trunk, and the limbs.

Bullous lesions, which may resemble erythema multiforme (Stevens–Johnson syndrome), may develop during the acute phase of measles.

7.15. B, C, D, and E.

Comment: In calcinosis cutis there are calcareous deposits in the skin alone.

The incidence of polyarthritis in psoriasis was estimated as 7% in one series (Ingram, 1954). Psoriatics with peripheral arthritis show a significant correlation with histocompatibility antigens B13 and BW17. If spondylitis is present there is a positive correlation with the presence of HLA B27.

Reiter's syndrome comprises a clinical triad of urethritis, conjunctivitis, and arthritis.

Albright's syndrome consists of café-au-lait patches, fibrous dysplasia of the long bones, and precocious puberty in girls.

7.16. A, B, and C.

Comment: Wood's light allows the emission of long-wave ultraviolet light (UVA), which shows a peak of 365 nm.

The treatment of choice for porphyria cutanea tarda (PCT) is regular venesection until a low serum iron level is induced. In PCT a simple screening test is Wood's light examination of the urine for coral-pink fluorescence. This is due to porphyrins present; in some instances it may also be seen in blister fluid *in situ*.

Tinea versicolor fluoresces pale yellow under Wood's light, which also helps to define unsuspected areas of infection.

7.17. B, D, and E.

Comment: In rosacea a variety of ocular complications may occur. These include the common blepharitis and conjunctivitis, the less common episcleritis and iritis, and the least common, but potentially blinding, keratitis.

Skin manifestations of Crohn's disease include erythema nodosum, erythema multiforme, and the rarer pyoderma gangrenosum. Conjunctivitis, uveitis, and iritis may also be associated features.

Behçet's syndrome is characterised by pyoderma, such as impetigo, folliculitis, cellulitis, acne-like lesions, and ulcers. Eye involvement is the most frequent cause of disability and common lesions are iridocyclitis and uveitis.

7.18. B, C, and D.

Comment: In general, immunisation is an elective procedure,which allows time to check that no contraindications exist prior to vaccination. Live vaccines should not be administered to pregnant women, because of the potential harm to the fetus. If there is a high risk of exposure to a potentially life-threatening disease, such as polio or yellow fever, the importance of vaccination may outweigh the possible risk to the fetus.

Live vaccines should not be given to patients who are receiving immunosuppressive therapy, including deep X-ray treatment, or to those who are suffering from lymphoma, leukaemia, Hodgkin's disease, or hypogammaglobulinaemia, in all of which the normal immunological system may be impaired.

Infantile eczema was an important contraindication to smallpox vaccination. Since the demise of smallpox, eczema should not be considered a contraindication to routine immunisation against diphtheria, tetanus, pertussis, or oral polio vaccines.

7.19. B, C, and D.

Comment: The erythrocyte sedimentation rate is elevated in 90% of patients with active systemic lupus erythematosus (SLE), but it does not correlate with disease activity or therapy, and it may be normal in the presence of florid SLE.

Rheumatoid factor is found in up to 40% of patients with SLE, but this is not a specific test and its presence does not appear to alter the course of the disease.

Positive antinuclear antibody tests are found in 98–99% of all patients with SLE. The antinuclear antibodies are most commonly IgG.

Retinal cytoid bodies are not specific to lupus erythematosus.

7.20. A, C, and D.

Comment: Systemic corticosteroids can substantially diminish the tuberculin reaction, as they suppress delayed hypersensitivity, the basis of the reaction.

A negative tuberculin test does not exclude *M. tuberculosis* infection, since 15% or more patients with proven tuberculosis may fail to react to 250 TU when first tested and may regain reactivity only as health returns.

Sarcoidosis, Hodgkin's disease, and viral exanthemata may produce false negative reactions. The tuberculin test may occasionally, but not frequently, be negative in old age or cachexia. If serious tuberculous infection is suspected it is wise to begin the test with 1:10000 old tuberculin (1 TU) to avoid necrosis at the injection site.

PAPER SEVEN

FURTHER READING

Alarçon-Segovia, D. (1961), Drug-induced lupus syndrome, *Mayo Clinic Proceedings*, **44**, 664.

Benedict, P.H., Szabo, G., Fitzpatrick, T.B., *et al.* (1968), Melanotic macules in Albright's syndrome and in neurofibromatosis, *Journal of the American Medical Association*, **205**, 618.

Bland, J.H., O'Brien, R., and Bouchard, R.E. (1958), Palmar erythema and spider angiomata in rheumatoid arthritis, *Annals of Internal Medicine*, **48**, 1026.

Calin, A., Fox, R., Gerber, D.J., and Gibson, D.S. (1978), The natural history of Reiter's syndrome, *Arthritis and Rheumatism*, **21**, 548.

Caplan, R.M. (1967), Medical uses of the Wood's lamp, *Journal of the American Medical Association*, **202**, 1035.

Christianson, H.B., Pankey, G.A., and Applewhite, M.L. (1968), Ulcers of skin due to *Brucella suis*, *Archives of Dermatology*, **98**, 175.

De Takats, G. and Fowler, E.F. (1962), Raynaud's phenomenon, *Journal of the American Medical Association*, **179**, 1.

Eddy, R.D., Ascheim, E., and Farber, E.M. (1964), Experimental analysis of isomorphic (Köebner) response in psoriasis, *Archives of Dermatology*, **89**, 579.

Estes, D. and Christian, C.L. (1971), The natural history of systemic lupus erythematosus by prospective analysis, *Medicine*, **50**, 85.

Fries, J.F. and Siegel, R.C. (1973), Testing the 'preliminary criteria for classification of SLE', *Annals of Rheumatic Diseases*, **32**, 171.

Goolamali, S.K. (1990), Management of acne vulgaris, *Prescriber's Journal*, **30**(2), 78.

Gowans, J.D.C. (1967), Reiter's syndrome, *Medical Science*, **39** (January).

Grigor, R., Edmonds, J., Lewkonia, R., *et al.* (1978), Systemic lupus erythematosus. A prospective analysis, *Annals of Rheumatic Diseases*, **37**, 121.

Harpey, J.P. (1973), Drugs and disseminated lupus erythematosus, *Adverse Drug Reaction Bulletin*, **43**.

Holti, G. (1965), The effect of intermittent low molecular dextran inffusions upon the digital circulation in systemic sclerosis, *British Journal of Dermatology*, 77, 560.

Ingram, J.T. (1954), The significance and management of psoriasis, *British Medical Journal*, ii, 823.

Lee, S.L. and Chase, P.H. (1975), Drug induced systemic lupus erythematosus: a critical review, *Seminars in Arthritis and Rheumatism*, 5, 83.

Leonard, D.G., O'Duffy, J.D., and Rogers, R.S. III (1978), Prospective analysis of psoriatic arthritis in patients hospitalised for psoriasis, *Mayo Clinic Proceedings*. 53, 511.

Luciano, A. and Rothfield, N.F. (1973), Patterns of nuclear fluorescence and DNA-binding activity, *Annals of Rheumatic Diseases*, **32**, 337.

Miller, D.L. (1964), Frequency of complications of measles, *British Medical Journal*, ii, 75.

Mills, O.H., Leyden, J.J., and Kligman, A.M. (1973), Tretinoin treatment of steroid acne, *Archives of Dermatology*, **108**, 381.

O'Duffy, J.D. (1977), Psoriatic arthritis, *Postgraduate Medicine*, **61**, 165.

Seville, R.H., Rao, P.S., Hutchinson, D.N., *et al.* (1970), Outbreak of Campbell de Morgan spots, *British Medical Journal*, i, 408.

Sherlock, S. and Scheuer, P.J. (1973), The presentation and diagnosis of 100 patients with primary biliary cirrhosis, *New England Journal of Medicine*, **289**, 674.

Stuart-Harris, C. (1975), The principles and practice of immunisation, *Practitioner*, **215**, 285.

Welliver, R.C., Cherry, J.D., and Holtzman, A.E. (1977), Typical, modified and atypical measles. An emerging problem in the adolescent and adult, *Archives of Internal Medicine*, **137**, 39.

PAPER EIGHT

8.1. A, C, and D.

Comment: In acquired syphilis a chancre develops at the site of inoculation after an incubation period that ranges from 10–90 days, with an average of 21 days. The chancre lasts from 1–5 weeks.

Non-treponemal serologic tests are usually negative until 2 weeks after the chancre has formed.

Secondary skin lesions appear 6–12 weeks after the onset of the chancre and may be seen before the chancre has disappeared.

Tertiary syphilis follows secondary syphilis and may persist for life, in an asymptomatic form, in 60–70% of patients, or it may progress to neurosyphilis (6.5%), cardiovascular disease (9.6%), or gumma formation (16%).

At present, the fluorescent treponeal antibody absorption (FTA-ABS) test is the most sensitive serological test for all stages of syphilis. Occasionally, false positive FTA-ABS reactions occur in healthy adults with no other evidence of syphilis, and many of these positives will revert to negative within a year.

8.2. A, B, C, and F.

Comment: Blue sclerae appear as such because of thinning of the sclera, which allows the pigment of the choroid to become apparent. In the Ehlers–Danlos syndrome ocular manifestations include blue sclerae, strabismus, and epicanthal folds.

Marfan's syndrome is an inherited disease of connective tissue. It is transmitted as an autosomal dominant trait; the most characteristic ocular change is dislocation of the lens (ectopia lentis), which is usually bilateral. Occasionally, blue sclerae are present.

Blue sclerae are the hallmark of osteogenesis imperfecta, a generalised connective tissue disorder which also involves the bones and skin. Common findings are multiple fractures and deformities, deafness due to otosclerosis, thin skin, lax joints, and hernias.

Ocular abnormalities are estimated to occur in 20–30% of patients with incontinentia pigmenti and include strabismus, nystagmus, cataracts, optic nerve atrophy, and blue sclerae.

Patients with Addison's disease develop hyperpigmentation of the conjunctiva.

Ocular complications in malaria include retinal haemorrhages, probably a result of secondary anaemia, and dendritic ulcers of the cornea due to associated herpes simplex infection.

8.3. A, B, C, D, E, and F.

Comment: Albinism is commonly inherited as an autosomal recessive trait. Ocular albinism, which shows no deficiency of cutaneous pigment, is inherited as a sex-linked recessive.

Six types of oculocutaneous albinism have been described, all of which have in common diminished or absent melanin in the skin, hair, and eyes, nystagmus, photophobia, and a decrease in visual acuity.

Tyrosinase positive and yellow mutant albinos have some capacity to tan, and their hair may yellow with age.

Albino skin is particularly predisposed to pre-cancerous keratoses and skin cancer, so effective protection against UVB (290–320 nm) is vital.

Photophobia is managed by avoiding the sun whenever possible, and by the use of a broad-brimmed hat and sunglasses.

8.4. A, B, C, and D.

Comment: The specific cutaneous lesions of leukaemia are morphologically identical to those of malignant lymphomas.

Chloroma, or granulocytic sarcoma, is a green tumour that is pathognomonic of leukaemia. It may arise with or precede the development of acute granulocytic leukaemia and is seen particularly in children and young adults. The term chloroma was adopted because the tumour forms a green colour due to the presence of the enzyme myeloperoxidase. The tumour develops from the infiltration of immature granulocytic cells within the periosteum, predominantly of the orbital and cranial bones.

Leukaemic infiltration of facial skin may simulate rosacea or lupus erythematosus.

Leukaemia cutis may be diagnosed by biopsy, but it is not always possible to identify the cell type with confidence.

8.5. B, C, D, and F.

Comment: Hereditary angioedema, a rare disorder, is inherited as an autosomal dominant trait. The onset is usually in early childhood; there are recurrent swellings of the skin and mucous membranes throughout life, often associated with vomiting and intestinal colic.

In systemic amyloidosis some one in four patients have skin lesions. Small papules, which may haemorrhage on firm stroking, occur on the scalp, face, lips, and tongue. Diffuse infiltration of the tongue may also occur and cause macroglossia. Facial plaques and oedematous stiffened fingers, as may be seen in systemic sclerosis, are other recognised forms of skin involvement. In some patients gastro-intestinal symptoms predominate.

In typhoid fever a variety of skin signs occur. The characteristic 'rose spots', which are pink papules that blanch on pressure, usually appear within 10 days of untreated illness. They are not tender and occur in crops, commonly over the abdomen. The face is almost never affected. Each crop lasts for 3–5 days, and they often continue to develop for 2–3 weeks. They heal without pigmentation. Erythema nodosum and urticarial lesions have also been noted with typhoid, and a 'telogen effluvium' and nail changes – Beau's lines – can occur as sequelae. Miliaria crystallina is very common, but in spite of the high fever of typhoid herpes labialis is exceedingly uncommon.

8.6. A, B, C, D, and F.

Comment: Chloroquine produces a blue–black pigmentation of the nail beds, while other antimalarials may induce transverse bands of pigmentation on the nail or the nail bed.

In Kinnier Wilson's disease the half-moons (lunulae) go blue.

In vitamin B_{12} deficiency a deep brownish-black pigmentation of the nails and nail beds has been described.

Azure lunulae result from argyria.

8.7. B and D.

Comment: Pruritic grouped vesicles that simulate dermatitis herpetiformis (DH) over the extensor surfaces or are scattered over the body have been seen with cancer. Choriocarcinoma and malignant tumours of the breast, bladder, ovary, prostate, rectum, and uterus have been reported with a DH-like eruption. In some, the eruption disappears after appropriate treatment of the underlying cancer. Erythema multiforme may also occur with neoplasia or with leukaemia and lymphomas.

Papular urticaria is a synonym for insect bites.

Epidermolysis bullosa refers to a group of disorders in which blisters form after minor trauma. Six varieties are inherited as autosomal dominant and two as autosomal recessive traits. In the so-called 'acquired' form there is no evidence of genetic inheritance, but several diseases have been associated with it. These include inflammatory bowel disease, diabetes mellitus, tuberculosis, carcinoma of the lung, and multiple myeloma. The association with carcinoma is therefore not a significant one.

8.8. B, C, and E.

Comment: The syndrome is transmitted as an autosomal dominant trait with a high degree of penetrance.

The vast majority (98%) have pigmentation (brown–black lentigines) of the lips, especially of the lower lip, and virtually 90% of patients also show pigmentation of the buccal mucosa. Less frequently, there is pigmentation of the palate and gingiva.

The pigment over the lips may fade with time, but that over the buccal mucosa does so less quickly and so aids diagnosis.

The syndrome comprises pigmentation with intestinal polyps, although occasionally there may be pigmentation alone. Polyps may be found anywhere in the mucus-secreting section of the gastro-intestinal tract, but are seen most commonly in the jejunum. They may be responsible for intussusception with intestinal obstruction, colic, melaena, or rectal bleeding.

8.9. B, D, and F.

Comment: Hyperhidrosis is a feature of thyrotoxicosis. At normal room temperatures this may not always be apparent, although one study showed that at an environmental temperature of 34°C, thyrotoxic patients produced significantly more sweat than did normal subjects.

In mucoviscidosis, or fibrocystic disease of the pancreas, concentrations of sodium and chloride in the sweat are significantly elevated; the demarcation may not be so clear in adults as in children, in whom a sodium concentration greater than 70 mmol/l of sweat is considered diagnostic.

Increased sweat and acrocyanosis are constant features of familial dysautonomia (Riley–Day syndrome), which also consists of an absence of tears associated with a relative indifference to pain, which in turn may cause Charcot joints.

Lesions of the hypothalamus often result in anhidrosis. Surgery on the hypothalamus or floor of the third ventricle may result in pyrexia due to thermoregulatory dysfunction.

8.10. B, C, E, and F.

Comment: Adenoma sebaceum, in essence angiofibromas, usually appear between 4–10 years of age and increase in number at puberty. The earliest cutaneous manifestations of tuberous sclerosis are hypomelanotic macules, the so-called ash-leaf spots, found on the trunk and limbs. They are best seen with Wood's light, which is absorbed by melanin and so outlines hypomelanotic areas well.

Fibromata also occur around the nail folds and, if large, may distort nail growth. They commonly appear at puberty and also increase in size with age.

Epilepsy is usually evident in the first 3 years of life, often in the form of infantile spasms, and is associated with mental retardation.

'Phakoma' (literally 'mother-spot') presents as a grey or yellow plaque in the retina in about 50% of cases.

Renal tumours, found in some 40% of cases, are usually benign hamartomas of the mixed type (angiomyolipomas). Malignant change occurs rarely.

Approximately 65% of patients have cyst-like areas in the phalanges.

8.11. A, B, D, E, and F.

Comment: The carcinoid syndrome is characterised by facial flushing, often of sudden onset. It is often accompanied by facial and periorbital oedema, as well as pulmonary and gastro-intestinal symptoms.

In Chagas' disease, or American trypanosomiasis, Romana's sign is present in half the patients in the acute phase. This is a unilateral, firm, violaceous oedema of the eyelids, frequently associated with conjunctivitis.

Trichinosis causes periorbital oedema, pyrexia, myalgia, and an eosinophilia. Bilateral orbital oedema and subungual and subconjunctival haemorrhages occurring in the first two weeks of illness are typical.

8.12. A, C, D, E, and F.

Comment: There have been numerous studies of human leucocyte antigens (HLAs) in Hodgkin's disease. Although no striking HLA frequency has been shown, subgroups of patients have been identified. An increased frequency of B8 occurred in those whose disease had a duration greater than 5 years, as well as in those with the lymphocytic type, while there was an increase in A1 in those with the mixed-cell type.

Numerous studies have shown no consistent association between an HLA and malignant melanoma.

Coeliac disease, in essence a gluten-sensitive enteropathy, is significantly associated with HLA B8. The antigen was found in 60–65% of children and 80–85% of adults with coeliac disease, suggesting a relationship between antigen and age of onset of the disease.

Sjögren's syndrome consists of the combination of keratoconjunctivitis sicca, xerostomia, and rheumatoid arthritis; it is termed such when any two of these features are present. There is an increased frequency of the antigen B8.

The primary antigen shown to occur with increased frequency in Behçet's disease is B5. This occurs more commonly in Caucasians and in the Japanese. In one study the frequency of B5 was 84.6% of 26 patients, compared with 25.3% in 138 controls.

An increased frequency of the antigen A10 has been found in pemphigus vulgaris.

8.13. B, D, and F.

Comment: L'eruption fixé – the 'fixed' drug eruption – recurs in the same site or sites each time the drug is administered. The reaction typically occurs as a well-defined circular or oval erythematous plaque, which turns brown in time. With repeated attacks existing lesions increase in size and new lesions appear. The lesions may appear anywhere on the body, although the lips, hands, and glans penis are commonly affected.

As well as being caused by quinine, sulphonamides, and phenolphthalein, fixed eruptions may also be brought on by barbiturates, oxyphenbutazone, and chlordiazepoxide.

Phenolphthalein is considered a safe and reliable drug and hence is found in proprietary purgatives; because it is tasteless it is included in those purgatives sold in the form of chewing gum or chocolate.

8.14. A, B, C, D, E, and F.

Comment: McCune–Albright's syndrome consists of patchy pigmentation, cystic bone lesions, and sexual precocity in girls.

The pigmentation consists of café-au-lait spots, often in a linear distribution and usually over the neck, sacrum, and buttocks. They tend to develop over the affected bones.

Bone involvement is commonly unilateral, with the femur and pelvis usually involved.

The sexual precocity noted in some females is not associated with demonstrable follicle-stimulating hormone or ovulation.

The disease usually becomes apparent between 5–15 years of age, often because of a pathological fracture.

The syndrome may be associated with hyperthyroidism, hyperparathyroidism, or gigantism.

8.15. B, C, D, and E.

Comment: The type of carcinoma that is induced by irradiation is, to some extent, dependent on the site damaged. Basal cell carcinomas (BCCs) are common following radiation to the face, scalp, and trunk, whereas squamous cell carcinomas are common on the hands. Radiation-induced BCCs of the scalp have been reported 20–25 years after X-ray treatment of the scalp for ringworm infection.

In most patients with xeroderma pigmentosum, fibroblasts lack the ability to repair ultraviolet light damage to DNA. This results in the early development of keratoses and skin carcinomata, predominantly on light-exposed skin.

Lupus vulgaris (cutaneous tuberculosis) usually occurs on the face and neck. Squamous cell and, occasionally, basal cell carcinoma may occur in lupus vulgaris as early as after 2 years, although usually not until after 10 or more years of the disease.

8.16. A, C, D, E, and F.

Comment: Urticaria may be provoked by a number of unrelated conditions. Dental caries, as a site of focal sepsis, may cause urticaria, as may other infections, such as hepatitis, Candida infection, or helminth infection in the gut or tissues.

Very occasionally, carcinoma may be the underlying cause and urticaria has been reported with carcinoma of the rectum and choriocarcinoma.

Urticaria has also been found in systemic lupus erythematosus (SLE, 7–22% of cases) and, uncommonly, chronic urticaria may be a presenting feature of SLE.

8.17. A, B, C, D, F, and G.

Comment: Two recessive and two dominant forms of pseudoxanthoma elasticum (PXE) are recognised. The earliest histological change in PXE is calcification of elastic fibres. Raised lysine and hydroxylysine levels in collagen have been found. The skin shows yellow flat papules, especially over the neck, axillae, elbows, and groin. With time, the skin becomes inelastic and redundant and may hang in folds.

Brownish streaks, which resemble vessels (hence angioid), occur in the fundus in over 85% of cases and are, in essence, breaks in the elastic tissue of Bruch's membrane.

Angioid streaks also occur in Paget's disease of bone, sickle cell anaemia, and the Ehlers–Danlos syndrome.

Retinal haemorrhage from damaged vessels is a serious risk.

By the third decade there may be absence of pulses in the arms and legs, associated with intermittent claudication in some.

Hypertension secondary to renal artery involvement occurs in 20% of patients.

Gastro-intestinal haemorrhage may be the presenting sign in an unsuspected case.

8.18. B, C, D, and F.

Comment: The presence of a thrombus in a vein is referred to as thrombophlebitis. Trauma to the vessel wall, leading to stasis and venous distension, as with bone fractures, is a well-recognised cause.

Debility, cachexia, and prolonged immobilisation also cause venous stasis, with slowing of the blood flow because of loss of the normal pumping action of the calf muscles. These are therefore more likely to induce venous thrombosis, especially in the older age group.

With a history of pulmonary embolism there is an increased risk of stasis-related or other forms of venous thrombosis; however, this is not a cause, but often a result of thrombophlebitis.

Cancer of the pancreas, in particular, may present as a 'migratory superficial thrombophlebitis', although cancers of the lung, stomach, or prostate may also do so.

An increased incidence of thrombophlebitis has also been associated with ulcerative colitis, prolonged administration of large doses of oestrogen, including and especially the oestrogen-containing contraceptive 'pill'.

8.19. A, B, C, D, and F.

Comment: In one study skin lesions were found to precede arthritis in 65%, arthritis antedated the psoriasis in 19%, and skin and joint involvement occurred virtually together in 16% of cases.

Five subgroups of psoriatic arthritis are recognised: the classic form, which affects the distal interphalangeal joints; peripheral mono or asymmetrical oligoarthritis; rheumatoid-like rheumatoid factor negative variety; arthritis mutilans; and, finally, the predominantly axial form – spondylitis and/or sacro-iliitis.

Psoriasis of the nails occurs in some 75% of patients with arthritis – the distal and mutilating forms of arthritis are especially associated with severe nail dystrophy.

Inflammatory eye lesions are common with conjunctivitis (the most frequent, 20%), uveitis (10%), and episcleritis (2%).

8.20. A, B, C, E, and F.

Comment: Generalised pruritus may be the sole manifestation of Hodgkin's disease years before other features of the disease become obvious.

Acquired ichthyosis also occurs and may clear when the lymphoma enters a remission. The ichthyosis varies from generalised dry skin to morphological changes in the skin that are indistinguishable from ichthyosis vulgaris, with its fish-like scales.

Exfoliative dermatitis may occasionally be the only feature of Hodgkin's disease for years before lymphadenopathy or visceral involvement become apparent. Commonly, however, exfoliative dermatitis is a result of a drug reaction or an exacerbation of a pre-existing dermatosis, such as eczema, psoriasis, or seborrhoeic dermatitis.

Hyperpigmentation develops in 10–30% of patients with Hodgkin's disease. It may be generalised or Addisonian in distribution. The pathogenesis is poorly understood.

Jaundice may result from lymphomatous infiltration of the liver and from biliary obstruction due to locally enlarged lymph nodes.

PAPER EIGHT

FURTHER READING

Allen, J.A., Lowe, D.C., Roddie, I.C., *et al*. (1973), Studies on sweating in clinical and experimental thyrotoxicosis, *Clinical Science and Molecular Medicine*, **45**, 765.

Almeyda, J. (1972), Epidermolysis associated with neoplasm of the bronchus, *British Journal of Dermatology*, **87**, 70.

Baker, S.J., Ignatius, M., Johnson, S., *et al*. (1963), Hyperpigmentation of skin: a sign of vitamin B_{12} deficiency, *British Medical Journal*, **1**, 1713.

Brunt, P.W. and McKusick, V.A. (1970), Familial dysautonomia. A report of genetic and clinical studies with a review of the literature, *Medicine*, **49**, 343.

Burns, R.E. (1975), Spontaneous revision of FTA–ABS test reactions, *Journal of the American Medical Association*, **234**, 617.

Clark, E.G. and Danbolt, N. (1964), The Oslo study of the natural course of untreated syphilis, *Medical Clinics of North America*, **48**, 613.

Eddy, D.D. and Farber, E.M. (1962), Pseudoxanthoma elasticum. Internal manifestations: a report of cases and a statistical review of the literature, *Archives of Dermatology*, **86**, 729.

Editorial (1981), Recurrent urticaria, *Lancet*, ii, 235.

Emmerson, R.W. (1975), Multicentric pigmented Bowen's disease of the perineum, *Proceedings of the Royal Society of Medicine*, **68**, 345.

Falchuk, Z.M., Rogentine, G.N., and Strober, W. (1972), Predominance of histocompatibility antigen HL-A8 in patients with gluten-sensitive enteropathy, *Journal of Clinical Investigation*, **51**, 1602.

Falk, J. and Osoba, D. (1971), HL-A antigens and survival in Hodgkin's disease, *Lancet*, ii, 1118.

Fitzpatrick, T.B., Szabo, G., Hori, Y., *et al*. (1968), White leaf shaped macules, earliest visible sign of tuberous sclerosis, *Archives of Dermatology*, **98**, 1.

Fitzpatrick, T.B. and Quevedo, W.C., Jr (1972), Albinism, In *The Metabolic Basis of Inherited Disease*, 3rd edn, Stanbury, J.B., Syngaarden, J.B., and Fredrickson, D.S. (Eds), McGraw-Hill, New York, p. 326.

Goodman, R.M., Smith, E.W., Paton, D., *et al*. (1963), Pseudoxanthoma elasticum: a clinical and histopathological study, *Medicine*, **42**, 297.

Gershwin, M.E., Terasaki, P.I., Graw, R., *et al*. (1975), Increased frequency of HL-A8 in Sjögren's syndrome, *Tissue Antigens*, **6**, 342.

Holt, J.F. and Dickerson, W.W. (1952), The osseus lesions of tuberous sclerosis, *Radiology*, **58**, 1.

Jarnum, S. (1965), Gastrointestinal haemorrhage and protein loss in primary amyloidosis, *Gut*, **6**, 14.

Katz, R.J., Dahl, M.V., Penneys, N., *et al.* (1973), HL-A antigens in pemphigus, *Archives of Dermatology*, **108**, 53.

Koplon, B.S. (1966), Azure lunulae due to argyria, *Archives of Dermatology*, **94**, 33.

Lambert, J.R. and Wright, V. (1976), Eye inflammation in psoriatic arthritis, *Annals of Rheumatic Disease*, **35**, 354.

Moll, J.M.H. and Wright, V. (1973), Psoriatic arthritis, *Seminars in Arthritis and Rheumatism*, **3**, 55.

Monroe, E.W. (1981), Urticaria, *International Journal of Dermatology*, **20**, 32.

Rubins, J. (1978), Cutaneous Hodgkin's disease, *Cancer*, **42**, 1219.

Skog, E. (1964), Cutaneous manifestations associated with internal malignant tumours with particular reference to vesicular and bullous lesions, *Acta Dermatovenereologica*, **44**, 114.

Sneddon, I. (1955), Acquired ichthyosis in Hodgkin's disease, *British Medical Journal*, i, 763.

Stokes, P.L., Holmes, G.K.T., Asquita, P., *et al.* (1973), Histocompatibility antigens associated with adult coeliac disease, *Lancet*, ii, 162.

Tobias, N. (1951), Dermatitis herpetiformis associated with visceral malignancy, *Urologic and Cutaneous Review*, **55**, 352.

Tuffanelli, D., Abraham, R., and Dubois, E.I. (1963), Pigmentation from antimalarial therapy, *Archives of Dermatology*, **88**, 419.

Witkop, C.J., Jr, Hill, C.W., Desnick, S., *et al.* (1973), Ophthalmologic, biochemical, platelet and ultrastructural defects in the various types of oculocutaneous albinism, *Journal of Investigative Dermatolgy*, **60**, 443.

PAPER NINE

9.1. A, C, D, F, and G.

Comment: Congenital hypothyroidism, or cretinism, produces a facies not easily missed. The features include widely set eyes with periorbital swelling, a broad flat nose, a large protruding tongue, dry skin, and sparse scalp hair.

The approximate frequency of Down's syndrome or mongolism is one in 1000 live births. The facies consists of low-set ears, with the eyes slanting upward because of the presence of a medial epicanthal fold. The bridge of the nose is generally poorly developed or absent. The tongue is usually enlarged and heavily fissured, and protrudes through the mouth, which tends to hang open.

In myasthenia gravis, weakness of the ocular muscles occurs and the eyelids droop. When there is facial involvement a relatively immobile facies results. The smile resembles a snarl because the lips elevate, but do not retract.

The most consistent sign of Wilson's disease, or hepatolenticular degeneration, is the pigmentation of the corneal margins, known as the Kayser-Fleischer ring. The pigmentation is either a golden brown or a green–brown and forms because of the deposition of copper in Descemet's membrane at the periphery of the cornea.

9.2. A, B, D, E, and F.

Comment: To date, eight varieties of the Ehlers–Danlos (ED) syndrome have been described on the basis of clinical and biochemical criteria. The various syndromes share certain features, including hyperextensible joints, fragile skin, poor wound healing, and easy bruising. Four of the eight types of Ehlers–Danlos syndrome (ED 1, 2, 3, and 8) are inherited as an autosomal dominant trait, three (ED 4, 6, and 7) as an autosomal recessive trait, and one (ED 5) as an X-linked recessive trait. In ED 3, unlike the other types, skin features are minimal.

In general joint dislocations are common and congenital dislocation of the hip is a frequent occurrence.

Umbilical, hiatal, and inguinal hernias are also common. Easy bruising occurs because of fragile blood vessels and poor connective tissue. There is no abnormality of the clotting mechanism.

9.3. A, B, C, D, E, and F.

Comment: Acanthosis nigricans is recognised for its association with abdominal cancer (80–90%) in adults. The commonest internal malignancy is a gastric carcinoma. It presents as warty or velvety hyperpigmented skin, commonly over the neck and flexures.

It may be inherited as an autosomal dominant trait or it may occur with simple obesity.

It has also been reported with a number of endocrinopathies, including acromegaly, Cushing's syndrome, diabetes mellitus, hypothyroidism, and hyperthyroidism.

Acanthosis nigricans may precede malignancy, sometimes by several years, although commonly the cancer and the acanthosis appear together.

9.4. B, C, E, and F.

Comment: Carcinoid tumours usually occur in the gastro-intestinal tract and produce serotonin, histamine, prostaglandins, and kinins.

A pellagra-like rash occurs because of a niacin deficiency which, it is believed, occurs because dietary tryptophan is utilised in serotonin formation.

Cardiac involvement, when present, is predominantly right-sided; right-sided heart failure is a serious problem and a common cause of death.

Carcinoid tumours of the appendix do not produce skin changes. When skin signs are present they indicate either liver metastases or a tumour whose blood supply does not drain into the portal system.

9.5. B, C, D, and E.

Comment: The basic defect in Hartnup's disease, inherited as an autosomal recessive trait, appears to be a failure of absorption of tryptophan from the gastro-intestinal tract and the renal tubule.

The rash is identical to that in pellagra and is believed to occur for similar reasons, i.e. a niacin deficiency. The eruption typically occurs over light-exposed areas and, although eczema-like to begin with, it heals with scaling and hyperpigmentation.

Temporary cerebellar ataxia, with nystagmus and hyperactive deep tendon reflexes, is a recognised feature of the disease.

Urinary chromatogram shows aminoaciduria, which is a persistent finding and does not improve with therapy.

9.6. B, C, D, E. and F.

Comment: Delay in the development of cutaneous metastases (5 or more years) has been noted not only in breast cancer, but also with treated cancers of the kidney, colon, ovary, and bladder.

Skin metastases, however, signify an extremely poor prognosis and the patient often dies within 3–6 months of their onset.

The scalp is a favourite site for metastases from the lung, the breast, and the genito-urinary tract. Loss of hair, resembling alopecia areata or scarring alopecia, may be the presenting sign.

Prostatic cancer may produce skin metastases in a zoster-like distribution over the flank because of perineural lymphatic spread.

9.7. A, C, and E.

Comment: Hair growth is normally divided into three stages: telogen, when the hair is resting; anagen, when it is actively growing; and catagen, when it is involuting. In the adult approximately 85% of the scalp hair is in anagen, 14% in telogen, and 1% in catagen.

With hair loss associated with the contraceptive pill, the telogen hairs are shed – a phenomenon known as telogen effluvium. Acute disease or emotional stress may provoke a similar hair loss.

With cyclophosphamide therapy some anagen follicles enter catagen prematurely and inhibition of mitosis results in a constriction of the hair shaft. These hairs may be shed 4–6 days after the first effective dose.

Heparin induces hair loss by shunting anagen follicles into telogen. The hair loss occurs 2–3 months after starting anticoagulant therapy. Phenytoin or diphenylhydantoin, an anti-epilepsy drug, induces hirsutism.

9.8. B, C, D, and E.

Comment: Mycosis fungoides is an uncommon disorder caused by T-lymphocyte proliferation. It is commoner in men and usually occurs in the 40–60-year-old group.

Pruritus associated with an eczematous or psoriasiform eruption may herald mycosis fungoides.

The disease may be confined to the skin for several years, but in two out of three patients there is spread to the lymph nodes.

Post-mortem findings have shown visceral involvement also, with the lung, liver, and spleen commonly affected.

Tests for delayed hypersensitivity and humoral antibody are normal in early disease, but in the late stages there may be impairment of cell-mediated hypersensitivity.

9.9. B, C, D, and E.

Comment: In acute and chronic lymphatic leukaemia specific cutaneous lesions usually involve the face and extremities.

In myeloid (granulocytic) leukaemia the trunk is commonly affected and in monocytic leukaemia a generalised eruption is typical.

Hyperkeratosis of the palms and soles – keratoderma or tylosis – occasionally associated with oesophageal cancer, has been reported in leukaemia.

Leukaemic infiltrates can appear in scars from recent surgery, trauma, burns, and herpes zoster.

In chronic lymphatic leukaemia, in particular, infiltration of the facial skin can be so severe as to produce a leonine facies.

9.10. A, C, D, and E.

Comment: In obstructive liver disease the pruritus is thought to correlate with changes in the ratio of dihydroxy bile salts (deoxycholate and chenodeoxycholate) to trihydroxy salts (cholates).

Cholestyramine, which tends to bind dihydroxy salts preferentially, relieves the pruritus in many patients.

Cholestyramine has also been found useful in the pruritus of polycythaemia rubra vera, although the mechanism for its beneficial action remains unexplained.

Thyrotoxicosis can present with pruritus, although in less than 10% of cases, and, if associated with palmar erythema and hyperpigmentation, may be confused with liver disease. The pruritus has been noted to subside once the thyroid 'state' has been brought under control.

9.11. B, C, D, and F.

Comment: Telangiectasia in hereditary haemorrhagic telangiectasia (HHT), or Rendu–Weber–Osler disease, is seen most commonly on the face and, specifically, on the nasal mucosa, the lips, and over the cheeks.

Anaemia is usually a result of recurrent bleeding from telangiectasia in the nasal mucosa and the gastro-intestinal tract. These haemorrhages, often spontaneous, become more frequent with time.

Pulmonary arteriovenous fistulae may develop and can cause clubbing and cyanosis.

Duodenal ulcer is not uncommonly associated with HHT and, in those with proven gastro-intestinal bleeding, the incidence has approached virtually 20% of patients.

9.12. A, B, C, and D.

Comment: Hepatic porphyria includes the acute intermittent variety (AIP), porphyria variegata, and porphyria cutanea tarda (PCT).

Barbiturates, sulphonamides, oestrogen, and the oral contraceptives may provoke an attack of abdominal pain, vomiting, and neuropsychiatric illness in AIP.

In porphyria variegata the same drugs may cause both cutaneous – photosensitivity with blistering – and abdominal symptoms similar to AIP. Griseofulvin and methyldopa are also recognised as drugs to be avoided in porphyria variegata.

In PCT barbiturates and sulphonamides have no deleterious effect, but oestrogens and chloroquine can.

9.13. A, C, D, and F.

Comment: Rickets in children causes frontal bossing and abnormal parietal bone flattening. Widening of sutures may also occur.

In late congenital syphilis, defined as congenital syphilis that has remained untreated until 2 years of age, frontal bossing, saddle nose, and a poorly developed maxilla are characteristic stigmata.

Pierre Robin syndrome is typified by micrognathia and a high arched or cleft palate. The tongue, although normal in size, tends to fall back, because of the ill-developed mandible, and obstruct the pharynx.

Paget's disease of bone is not a disease of children; it has been estimated to occur in some 3% of individuals over 40 years old.

9.14. B, C, D, E, and F.

Comment: Achalasia is not associated with skin disease.

Candidiasis may involve both the skin and the oesophagus; the radiological appearances in the latter may resemble those of oesophageal varices. Systemic sclerosis affects only the lower two-thirds of smooth muscle portion of the oesophagus, leaving normal contractions in the upper third. Skin signs are invariably present.

In Chagas'disease, caused by *Trypanosoma cruzi*, there is dilatation and impaired peristalsis of the oesophagus or colon. In the acute phase an inoculation 'chagoma' may form on the face or arms, and marks the site of the insect vector bite. This heals with pigmentation. Morbilliform or urticarial lesions may also occur during the course of the disease.

9.15. A, B, D, and F.

Comment: Infectious mononucleosis and cytomegalovirus mononucleosis both cause a febrile illness associated with headache, myalgia, and sore throat. Rubella-like rashes, lasting a day or two, occur, but when ampicillin is prescribed as treatment an extensive erythematous eruption, which tends to be prolonged, follows. In one study (Shapiro *et al.*, 1969) a rash was reported in 9.5% of 422 patients treated with ampicillin, in 4.5% of 622 patients treated with other penicillins, and in 1.8% of 2941 patients who did not receive either of these drugs.

The incidence of ampicillin rashes has also been greater in patients with viral infections than in those with other infections.

9.16. A, B, C, D, and E.

Comment: Dapsone is valuable in the treatment of all types of leprosy and in suppressing the rash of dermatitis herpetiformis. It is also of value in toxoplasmosis and mycetoma and, when combined with other antimalarials, in the prophylaxis of malaria.

Methaemoglobinaemia is occasionally seen and, if severe, may warrant therapy with methylene blue administered intravenously.

Dapsone is known to induce haemolytic anaemia, particularly in subjects with glucose-6-phosphate dehydrogenase deficiency, an abnormality common in West African, Middle Eastern, Mediterranean, and Southern Chinese peoples.

Peripheral neuropathy appears to be dose-related and usually resolves on reduction of the dose or discontinuation of the drug.

9.17. A, B, C, and D.

Comment: Erythema nodosum is a common skin manifestation of ulcerative colitis in children. Pyoderma gangrenosum is another, but both these occur in less than 5% of patients.

Secondary syphilitic eruptions may present in a number of ways, one of which is a pityriasis rosea-like eruption. Differentiating points are that the syphilitic eruption lacks the 'Christmas-tree' pattern of pityriasis rosea and that it also affects the palms and soles, which pityriasis rosea does not.

Atopic eczema in children may cause keratoconus, which is thought to result from persistent rubbing of the eyelids. Cataracts occur in 5–10% of adults with severe atopic eczema, but are rare in children.

9.18. A, C, D, and E.

Comment: The lesions of chickenpox first appear on the trunk and scalp and are usually associated with pyrexia, malaise, and myalgia. The presenting macular lesions rapidly pass through the stages of papules, vesicles, pustules, and crust formation.

The virus is readily cultured from vesicle fluid.

As the rash appears in crops there are lesions in different stages in the same anatomical area, a useful diagnostic sign.

Varicella may be complicated by meningoencephalitis, myocarditis, hepatitis, nephritis, and orchitis.

9.19. A, B, C, E, and F.

Comment: Lepromatous leprosy is characterised by a negative lepromin test, which confirms decreased resistance. Skin lesions consist of macules, plaques, and papulo-nodules (lepromas). The latter are seen commonly on the ears, face, elbows, knees, and buttocks.

Lupus pernio, one of the cutaneous markers of sarcoid, is a persistent violaceous lesion with a predilection for the nose, cheeks, and ears. It is often found with sarcoid of the upper respiratory tract.

Chondrodermatitis helicis nodularis produces a painful nodule on the helix. The nodule may interfere with sleep, as lying on it can be intensely painful. The pain may also be triggered off by cold.

Lupus vulgaris, or post-primary cutaneous tuberculosis, occurs in patients with a high degree of tuberculin sensitivity. A common form of tuberculosis some 25 years ago, its incidence has declined over the years. It usually occurs on the head or neck and often starts on the nose or cheek. The earlobes are frequently affected.

9.20. A, C, D, E, and F.

Comment: Infestation with *Enterobius vermicularis* (threadworm) was found to be the cause of pruritus vulvae in only 14 of 912 women in one study. In children it is more common and may present as a vulvovaginitis with dysuria or a yellow stain on the pants. To collect a specimen for threadworm ova, Sellotape is applied several times to the stretched perineal skin – ova will adhere to it. The collection is best made in the morning on awaking as the ova are laid overnight by the gravid female threadworm. The tape is then placed on a glass slide and examined under the microscope.

Pediculosis pubis, a common infection caused by the crab louse *Phthirius pubis,* causes intense pruritus vulvae. A successful treatment is the application of gammabenzene hexachloride.

Lichen sclerosus et atrophicus is a disease of unknown aetiology, predominantly of women, usually middle-aged or over, that invariably affects the genitalia. Persistent pruritus vulvae is a common symptom and responds to some extent to topical steroids.

Epithelioma of the vulva may also present with pruritus vulvae.

PAPER NINE

FURTHER READING
Barnes, H.M., Sarkaney, I, and Calnan, C.D. (1974), Pruritus and thyrotoxicosis, *St John's Hospital Dermatological Society*, **60**, 59.
Baron, D.N., Dent, C.E., Harris, H., *et al.* (1956), Hereditary pellagra-like skin rash with temporary cerebellar ataxia, constant renal amino-aciduria and other bizarre biochemical features, *Lancet*, **ii**, 421.
Beighton, P. (1970), *The Ehlers–Danlos Syndrome*, Heinemann, London.
Brownstein, M.H. and Helwig, E.B. (1973), Spread of tumours to the skin, *Archives of Dermatology*, **107**, 80.
Croydon, E.A.P., *et al.* (1973), Prospective study of ampicillin rash. Report of a collaborative study group, *British Medical Journal*, **i**, 7.
Epstein, E.H., Levin, D.L., Croft, J.G., Jr, *et al.* (1972), Mycosis fungoides. Survival, prognostic features, response to therapy and autopsy findings, *Medicine*, **51**, 61.

Flaxman, B.A. (1981), Pruritus: identifying and treating the causes, *Postgraduate Medicine*, **69**, 177.

Graham-Smith, D.D. (1970), The carcinoid syndrome, *Gut*, **11**, 189.

Härkonen, M. (1981), Hereditary hemorrhagic telangiectasia (Osler–Weber–Rendu disease) complicated by pulmonary arteriovenous fistula and brain abscess, *Acta Medica Scandinavica*, **209**, 137.

Isaacs, N.J. and Ertel, N.H. (1971), Urticaria and pruritus: uncommon manifestations of hyperthyroidism, *Journal of Allergy*, **48**, 73.

Jacobson, R.J. (1980), Polycythaemia vera: clinical features, differential diagnosis and treatment, *Primary Care*, **7**, 489.

Kounis, N.G. and Constantinidis, K. (1980), Lupus vulgaris: a rare dermal involvement, *Practitioner*, **224**, 1283.

Laranja, F.S., Dias, E., Nobrega, G., *et al.* (1956), Chagas' disease – a clinical, epidemiologic and pathologic study, *Circulation*, **14**, 1035.

Leading article (1975), Ampicillin rashes, *British Medical Journal*, ii, 708.

McKenzie, A.W. and Acharya, U. (1972), The oral contraceptive and variegate porphyria, *British Journal of Dermatology*, **86**, 453.

Moore, M.R. (1980), International review of drugs in acute porphyria – 1980, *International Journal of Biochemistry*, **12**, 1089.

Nordqvist, B.C. and Kinney, J.P. (1976), T- and B-cells and cell-mediated immunity in mycosis fungoides, *Cancer*, **37**, 714.

Pumpianski, R. and Sheskin, J. (1965), Pruritus vulvae: a five year survey, *Dermatologica*, **131**, 446.

Rajka, G. (Ed), (1975), *Atopic Dermatitis. Major Problems in Dermatology*, Vol. 3, W.B. Saunders, London.

Reingold, I.M. (1966), Cutaneous metastases from internal carcinoma, *Cancer*, **19**, 162.

Ridley, C.M. (1975), *The Vulva. Major Problems in Dermatology*, Vol. 5, W.B. Saunderws, London.

Shapiro, S., Slone, D., Siskind, V., *et al.* (1969), Drug rash with ampicillin and other penicillins, *Lancet*, ii, 969.

Stecker, R.H. and Lake, C.F. (1965), Hereditary haemorrhagic telangiectasia, *Archives of Otolaryngology*, **82**, 522.

Walton, J.N. (Ed), (1981), *Disorders of Voluntary Muscle*, 4th edn, Churchill Livingstone, Edinburgh.

Wheelock, M.C., Frable, W.J., and Urnes, P.D. (1962), Bizarre metastases from malignant neoplasms, *American Journal of Clinical Pathology*, **37**, 475.

Zelicovici, Z., Lahav, M., and Cahane, P. (1977), Pruritus as a presentation of myelomatosis, *British Medical Journal*, ii, 1154.

PAPER TEN

10.1. B, D, E, and F.

Comment: In psoriasis the epidermal turnover time is greatly increased and has been estimated at between 2–5 days, as compared with 27 days for normal epidermis. This increased epidermal proliferation results in the formation of thick loosely adherent silvery scales that overlie an erythematous lesion.

The nails also show changes, although these occur only in some 25–50% of patients. Subungual hyperkeratosis, punctate pitting, or onycholysis are the usual findings.

Oral lesions are rare in psoriasis vulgaris, although they have been seen in acute generalised pustular psoriasis as whitish non-ulcerated lesions on the tongue and rarely on the buccal mucosa.

10.2. A, B, C, D, and E.

Comment: Alkaptonuria is an inborn error of tyrosine metabolism. The absence of the enzyme homogentisic acid oxidase results in the accumulation of homogentisic acid in tissue. Freshly voided urine turns black on standing. Cutaneous manifestations include pigmented lesions on the sclerae and cartilage of the ears, as well as facial and flexural pigmentation. Black renal stones that contain calcium, phosphate, and oxalate have also been reported.

Sarcoidosis produces a variety of skin lesions – lupus pernio, erythema nodosum, and hypopigmented macules. Hypercalcaemia may be associated and cause renal calculi and nephrocalcinosis.

Henoch–Schönlein purpura is a common syndrome characterised by the acute onset of abdominal pain, arthralgia, and rash. Purpura may be the only sign. Renal involvement occurs in approximately 25% of patients and presents as haematuria and/or proteinuria.

In gout, tophi consisting of uric acid form especially on the ears, olecranon, and prepatellar bursae. The elevated serum uric acid may also cause renal calculi. Unlike systemic amyloidosis, primary cutaneous amyloidosis has no renal associations.

10.3. A, B, and C.

Comment: The Peutz–Jeghers syndrome consists of pigmented macules on the lips, face, buccal mucosa, and hands, which are associated with polyps that occur commonly in the jejunum and ileum.

Gardner's syndrome is characterised by multiple polyps of the small and large intestine, associated with osteomas and soft tissue lesions –

lipomas, fibromas, sebaceous cysts, and leiomyomas. Patients show an increased frequency of colorectal carcinoma.

In acute intermittent porphyria cutaneous lesions do not occur.

In the Plummer–Vinson syndrome there are no skin signs although koilonychia, as a result of hypochromic anaemia, may occur with an anterior oesophageal web.

10.4. A – 6, B – 4, C – 2, D – 5, E – 3, and F – 1.

10.5. A, B, C, and F.

Comment: In approximately 25% of patients with psoriasis there is a symmetrical arthritis indistinguishable, apart from the absence of rheumatoid factor, from rheumatoid arthritis. In this group there is a tendency to develop arthritis mutilans, with resorption of bone and telescoping of digits.

Arthritis is associated with ulcerative colitis in some 10% of patients. In 10% of these patients with arthritis, a pattern of disease like that of rheumatoid arthritis develops.

Patients with acromegaly develop degenerative joint disease akin to osteoarthritis. Increased growth hormone results in hypertrophy of bone and cartilage.

Classic haemophilia results from a deficiency of Factor VIII, essential in blood clotting. Haemorrhages into joints, especially of the elbows, knees, and ankles, are characteristic. The hands are usually spared. Repeated haemarthroses cause immobility and destruction of the joints.

10.6. A, B and F.

Comment: The Sturge–Weber syndrome is associated with a port-wine naevus, usually in the distribution of the trigeminal nerve which overlies a similar vascular malformation of the meninges. Calcification of the capillaries of the cortex produces the well-described 'tram-line' calcification.

Tuberous sclerosis, or epiloia, consists of several cutaneous signs. The one commonly referred to is facial hamartoma or adenoma sebaceum. Cerebral calcification may also be present.

Cysticercosis is caused by the larvae cysticercus cellulosae, of the adult pork tapeworm *Taenia solium*. The larvae invade several organs, but primarily the subcutaneous tissue where they induce an inflammatory reaction and eventually calcify. The cysts in the skin are usually asymptomatic and not clinically diagnostic. Cerebral lesions occur next in order of frequency and may simulate a tumour and cause epilepsy. Skull X-rays show calcified cysticerci.

In congenital toxoplasmosis cerebral calcification may occur several months after the initial presenting signs of epilepsy, hepatosplenomegaly, and a non-specific maculopapular rash.

In idiopathic hypoparathyroidism the nails show the characteristic friable, brittle distal area with irregular longitudinal grooves over the proximal nail. The skin is usually dry and body hair sparse. Calcification occurs in the basal ganglia.

10.7. A, B, C, D, E, F, and G.

Comment: Polyarteritis nodosa is a rare disease characterised by an arteritis of small- and medium-sized vessels, e.g. the size of the hepatic and coronary arteries. Infarcts in the skin may present as haemorrhagic bullae or purpura.

Tender subcutaneous nodules often occur in groups along the course of superficial arteries, particularly over the lower limbs.

Fever occurs at some stage in virtually all patients and may be part of the complex of presenting symptoms in some 50% of patients. The first description of the disease (Kussmaul and Maier, 1866) included fever, abdominal pain, tachycardia, and haematuria in a young man who died within a few months.

The arterial involvement in polyarteritis nodosa results in hypertension and its sequelae.

Abdominal pain may be a consequence of hepatic or splenic infarction or pancreatitis.

10.8. A, D, and F.

Comment: The hilar glands may be enlarged although not well demarcated in measles, pertussis, and varicella pneumonia. In varicella the pneumonia generally appears 1–6 days after the onset of the rash, the severity of which correlates well with the degree of lung involvement.

During the early phases of disease 10% of patients with infectious mononucleosis exhibit a rubella-like eruption on the trunk and extremities. Classically, it is provoked by ampicillin prescribed for the associated sore throat. Lymphadenopathy is the hallmark of infectious mononucleosis, but if hilar lymphadenopathy is seen on routine chest X-ray, it should be further investigated to exclude another cause.

Pulmonary lesions in sporotrichosis result from inhalation of the fungus *Sporothrix schenkii*. Two forms of pulmonary disease are described. The more common produces cavitation and resembles tuberculosis and the other, which is less chronic, is characterised by hilar lymphadenopathy and sparing of lung parenchyma.

10.9. B, C, D, and F.

Comment: In hypopituitarism the skin is smooth and pale. It often feels dry, due in part to decreased sebum production, and there may be premature wrinkling, seen best around the eyes. In addition, there may be a diffuse alopecia and scant body hair. Pituitary insufficiency causes short stature, although it is responsible for less than 10% of such cases.

Children with phenylketonuria typically have fair skin, blue eyes, blonde hair, and sunburn easily. Other cutaneous features are eczema and dermographism. The untreated phenylketonuric child develops mental and growth retardation.

Cushing's syndrome produces a variety of skin signs which include facial acne, plethora, hirsutes, striae, ecchymoses, and superficial fungal infection. Osteoblastic function is depressed by excess production of glucocorticoids and skeletal maturation in children may be significantly delayed.

10.10. B, C, D, E, and F.

Comment: Oesophageal involvement is common in systemic sclerosis. An incidence of 80% has been found using sensitive manometric techniques. Oesophageal dysfunction occurs because atrophy and fibrous tissue replace the smooth muscle normally present. Progressive dysphagia may occur because of impaired peristalsis in the lower half of the oesophagus, but it may also reflect the formation of an oesophageal stricture.

A hiatus hernia may be present in some 50% of patients.

Colonic involvement in systemic sclerosis usually occurs in association with small bowel disease. Radiologic features include loss of haustrations, wide-neck diverticulae (especially in the transverse and descending colon), and, with progressive disease, generalised dilatation of the colon. Well-defined 'honeycomb' shadows form part of the radiological appearance of fibrosing alveolitis, causes of which are systemic sclerosis and rheumatoid arthritis.

10.11. A, B, C, and E.

Comment: Neurofibromatosis shows an increased association with cystic lung disease. Irradiation of the thorax for therapeutic purposes, as for carcinoma of the breast, may induce fibrosis of underlying lung tissue. It may also cause atrophy and telangiectasia in the irradiated skin.

Lung lesions are seen commonly in sarcoidosis. There are four X-ray appearances recognised:

- Bilateral hilar and right paratracheal lymph node involvement.
- Persistence of lymph nodes with pulmonary infiltration.
- Pulmonary infiltration with no identifiable mediastinal lymphadenopathy.
- Fibrosis with bullae.

In dermatomyositis basal shadowing associated with other radiographic features of fibrosing alveolitis may occasionally be seen.

10.12. A, B, C, and D.

Comment: Glucocorticoids stimulate bone marrow, fat tissue, and hair; in Cushing's syndrome, hirsutism (usually without other signs of virilism), obesity, and polycythaemia are common findings.

Stein–Leventhal or the polycystic ovary syndrome results in hirsutism associated with amenorrhoea, infertility, and obesity.

The several varieties of congenital adrenal hyperplasia have in common an inborn error in cortisol synthesis with secondary overproduction of ACTH and steroids, with virilising and hypertension-inducing properties.

Arrhenoblastoma, an ovarian tumour, may contain testicular tissue. *In vitro* production of testosterone has been demonstrated in these tumours and hirsutism is a consequence of this.

In Sheehan's syndrome (post-partum necrosis of the pituitary gland) scalp hair becomes sparse and pubic and axillary hair are totally lost.

In dystrophia myotonica premature grey hair and male-pattern alopecia accompany myotonia and muscle wasting.

10.13. A, B, C, F, and G.

Comment: In porphyria cutanea tarda (PCT) bullae occur commonly over sites prone to trauma. The bullae, in both PCT and pemphigoid, are subepidermal in site. Histological examination of a blister in PCT shows little or no dermal inflammatory infiltrate.

Although uncommon, blisters may form one of the cutaneous signs of congenital syphilis. The bullae may be generalised, but have a predilection for the palms and soles. They vary in size from 1–5 cm diameter and may be associated with a maculopapulopustular eruption.

Scabies caused by the ubiquitous mite *Sarcoptes scabiei* typically induces pruritus which is worse at night. The lesions vary according to the degree of sensitisation of the host, with the pathognomonic lesion being the burrow, the home of the female mite. In adults vesicles develop, while in infants bullae may form, especially on the palms and soles.

10.14. B, C, D, and E.

Comment: Yellow nails are seen with the yellow-nail syndrome, in which lymphoedema, commonly of the lower limbs, pleural effusion, and bronchiectasis have been associated. Yellow nails may also occur rarely with prolonged tetracycline therapy.

Heliotrope (purplish-red) erythema around the eyes, but most marked on the upper lids, is characteristic of dermatomyositis. The eruption may also involve the forehead, the 'butterfly' area of the face, and the neck. As in systemic lupus erythematosus it may be initiated by ultraviolet light.

Dilated nail fold capillaries, or periungual telangiectasia, occur principally in dermatomyositis and systemic lupus erythematosus.

In the childhood or juvenile form of dermatomyositis, calcification in subcutaneous tissue and muscle is common. It may be found in more than 50% of children who survive the first 2 years of the disease. The overall incidence of calcinosis cutis varies between 10–20%.

Unlike systemic sclerosis the subcutaneous calcium deposits in dermatomyositis rarely form over the fingers.

10.15. B, C, and E.

Comment: Necrobiosis lipoidica diabeticorum (NLD) occurs three times more commonly in women.

The typical patch usually occurs on the shins, although lesions may form on the face, arms, and trunk.

The plaque commonly shows atrophy and telangiectasia and ulceration may occur spontaneously or as a result of trauma.

The treatment of NLD is unsatisfactory. Control of hyperglycaemia with insulin or oral hypoglycaemic agents does not alter the course of the necrobiotic plaques.

Necrobiosis may precede the development of diabetes mellitus, although it is usual for the diabetes to have been present for several years before the necrobiosis lipoidica becomes apparent.

10.16. B, C, D, E, and F.

Comment: Chickenpox may develop in those not previously exposed to the disease after exposure to a patient with herpes zoster. Previous chickenpox, but not herpes simplex infection, is the source of herpes zoster. The varicella virus spreads via sensory nerve fibres to sensory ganglia, where it lies dormant.

Reactivation of the virus may be induced by injection of arsenicals, immunosuppressive therapy (radiation, antimetabolites, steroids), local trauma, and the development of reticuloses or leukaemia.

In Hodgkin's disease, 20–50% of patients develop herpes zoster, with the highest incidence in those with advanced disease or receiving immunotherapy.

10.17. A – 5, B – 6, C – 1, D – 2, E – 4, and F – 3.

10.18. A, B, C, F, and G.

Comment: Serum levels of muscle enzymes reflect disease activity in dermatomyositis. Serum aldolase is considered the most sensitive, but the creatine phosphokinase level reflects muscle fibre damage more accurately and is probably the best index of disease activity. The lactic dehydrogenase and serum glutamic oxalacetic transaminase levels also rise with active myositis. Enzyme levels are usually decreased by steroid therapy, but may return to normal when severe muscle atrophy has developed.

The antinuclear antibody, when present in dermatomyositis, usually shows the less specific homogenous or speckled pattern.

Unlike in systemic lupus erythematosus, leucopenia is rare in dermatomyositis.

The 24-hour urinary creatine excretion in normal adults does not exceed 100 mg. Values greater than 200 mg/24 hours are suggestive of active disease.

Muscle biopsy remains the best single diagnostic test, especially when taken from an obviously weak or tender muscle.

10.19. B, C, E, and F.

Comment: The single constant symptom of dermatitis herpetiformis (DH) is a burning pruritus of variable degree. The pruritus increases with the development of skin lesions – scratching these often relieves the itch.

DH shows a 2:1 predominance of males.

Grouped vesicles occur in a symmetrical distribution and, if undisturbed, may reach a size of 1 cm or more in diameter.

Mucosal abnormalities of the jejunum are extremely common in DH. Total or partial villous atrophy occurs in 80% of patients.

Dapsone (diaminodiphenylsulphone) controls the pruritus and skin lesions within 24–48 hours. Relapse occurs equally quickly on withdrawal of the drug.

10.20. A, C, D and F.

Comment: Subacute bacterial endocarditis is associated with subungual (splinter) haemorrhages, conjunctival and palatal petechiae, tender spots (Osler's nodes), usually on the tips of the fingers and toes, and non-tender erythematous macules or nodules (Janeway's lesion) on the palms and soles.

Trichinosis is an infection caused by *Trichinella spiralis* found in inadequately cooked infected meat, commonly pork. During the course of the illness various cutaneous signs, including splinter haemorrhages, occur. The parasite may be found in biopsy specimens of the nail bed.

Arteritis in rheumatoid arthritis may present as small infarcts around the nails and splinter haemorrhages. Long-term corticosteroid therapy appears to predispose patients to vasculitic lesions.

PAPER TEN

FURTHER READING

Baum, G.L., Donnerberg, R.L., Stewart, D., *et al.* (1969), Pulmonary sporotrichosis, *New England Journal of Medicine*, **280**, 410.

Bongiovanni, A.M. and Root, A.W. (1963), The adrenogenital syndrome, *New England Journal of Medicine*, **268**, 1283.

Church, R.E. and Ellis, A.R.P. (1950), Cystic pulmonary fibrosis in generalised scleroderma: Report of two cases, *Lancet*, i, 392.

Coli, R.D., Moore, J.P., La Marche, P.H., *et al.* (1970), Gardner's syndrome: a revisit to a previously described family, *American Journal of Digestive Diseases*, **15**, 551.

Elder, G.H., Gray, C.H., and Nicholson, D.C. (1972), The porphyrias: a review, *Journal of Clinical Pathology*, **25**, 1013.

Ellis, K. and Renthal, G. (1962), Pulmonary sarcoidosis. Roentgenographic observations on the course of the disease, *American Journal of Roentgenology*, **88**, 1070.

Fisher, I. and Orkin, M. (1964), Cutaneous form of periarteritis nodosa – an entity? *Archives of Dermatology*, **89**, 180.

Hare, P.J. (1955), Necrobiosis lipoidica, *British Journal of Dermatology*, **67**, 365.

Hill, D.M., Rhodes, E.I., Sheldon, J., *et al.* (1966), Necrobiosis lipoidica. Serum insulin and prednisone–glycosuria tests in a non-diabetic group, *British Journal of Dermatology*, **78**, 332.

Kilpatrick, Z.M., Greenberg, P.A., and Sanford, J.P. (1965), Splinter haemorrhages – their clinical significance, *Archives of Internal Medicine*, **115**, 730.

Konstantinov, D. and Stanoeva, L. (1973), Persistent scabious nodules, *Dermatologica*, **147**, 321.

Laymon, C.W. (1953), Oochronosis, *Archives of Dermatology and Syphilology*, **67**, 553.

Lindgren, I. and Lundmark, C. (1956), Periarteritis nodosa as a skin disease, *Acta Dermatovenereologica*, **36**, 343.

McEwen, C. (1968), Arthritis complicating ulcerative colitis, *Clinics in Orthopaedics*, **59**, 9.

Muller, S.A., Winkelmann, R.K., and Brunsting, L.A. (1959), Calcinosis in dermatomyositis. Observations on course of disease in children and adults, *Archives of Dermatology*, **79**, 669.

Peachey, R.D.G., Creamer, B., Pierce, J.W., *et al.* (1969), Sclerodermatous involvement of the stomach and large bowel, *Gut*, **10**, 285.

Poirier, T.J. and Rankin, G.B. (1972), Gastrointestinal manifestations of progressive systemic sclerosis based on a review of 364 cases, *American Journal of Gastroenterology*, **58**, 30.

Rifkind, D. (1966), The activation of varicella-zoster virus infection by immunosuppressive therapy, *Journal of Laboratory and Clinical Medicine*, **68**, 463.

Rose, G.A. and Spencer, H. (1957), Polyarteritis nodosa, *Quarterly Journal of Medicine*, **27**, 43.

Savard, K., Gut, M., Dorfman, R.I., *et al.* (1961), Formation of androgens by human arrhenoblastoma tissue *in vitro*, *Journal of Clinical Endocrinology*, **21**, 165.

Schwarz, M., Mathau, R.A., Sadn, S.A., *et al.* (1975), Interstitial lung disease in polymyositis and dermatomyositis. Analysis of six cases and review of the literature, *Medicine*, **55**, 89.

Sokal, J.E. and Firat, D. (1965), Varicella-zoster infection in Hodgkin's disease, *American Journal of Medicine*, **39**, 452.

Van Scott, E.J. and Ekel, T.M. (1963), Kinetics of hyperplasia in psoriasis, *Archives of Dermatology*, **88**, 373.

White, D.K., Leiss, H.J., and Miller, A.S. (1976), Intraoral psoriasis associated with widespread dermal psoriasis, *Oral Surgery*, **41**, 174.

SELECTED BIBLIOGRAPHY

Braverman, I.M. (1981), *Skin Signs of Systemic Disease*, 2nd edn, W.B. Saunders, Philadelphia.

Champion, R.H., Burton, J.L., and Ebling, F.G.J. (Eds), (1992), *Rook, Wilkinson, Ebling Textbook of Dermatology*, 5th edn, Blackwell Scientific, Oxford.

Dudley Hart, F. (Ed.), (1985), *French's Index of Differential Diagnosis*, 12th edn, John Wright & Sons Ltd, Bristol.

Fitzpatrick, T.B., Eisen, A.Z., Wolff, K., *et al.* (Eds), (1979), *Dermatology in General Medicine*, 2nd edn, McGraw-Hill, New York.

Gorlin, R.J., Pindborg, J.J., and Cohen, M.M. (1976), *Syndromes of the Head and Neck*, 2nd edn, McGraw-Hill, New York.

Lebwohl, M. (Ed), (1988), *Difficult Diagnoses in Dermatology*, Churchill Livingstone, Edinburgh.

Scriver, C.B., Beaudet, A.L., Sly, W.S., and Valle, D. (Eds), (1989), *The Metabolic Basis of Inherited Disease*, 6th edn, McGraw-Hill, New York.

Wetherall, D.J., Ledingham, J.G.G., and Warrell, D.A. (Eds), (1987), *Oxford Textbook of Medicine*, 2nd edn, Oxford University Press, Oxford.

Wyngaarden, J.B. and Smith, L.H., Jr (Eds), (1988), *Cecil Textbook of Medicine*, 18th edn, W.B. Saunders, Philadelphia.

INDEX

Note: The index covers the comments and the entries are given by answer number.

142